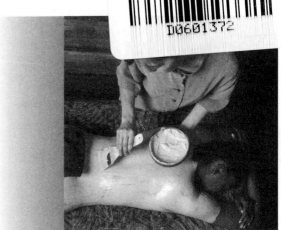

THE SPA
ENCYCLOPEDIA

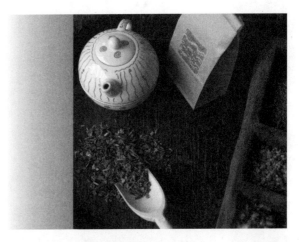

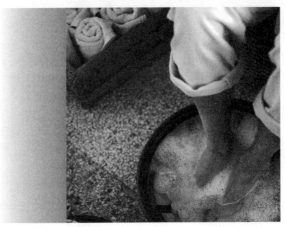

THE SPA
ENCYCLOPEDIA

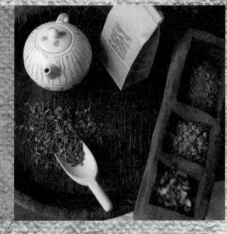

A Guide to
Treatments & Their
Benefits for
Health & Healing

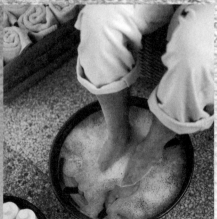

HANNELORE R. LEAVY
REINHARD R. BERGEL, PhD

THOMSON
™
DELMAR LEARNING

Australia Canada Mexico Singapore Spain United Kingdom United States

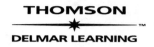

THOMSON
TM
DELMAR LEARNING

The Spa Encyclopedia:
A Guide to Treatments & Their Benefits for Health & Healing
Hannelore R. Leavy and Reinhard R. Bergel, PhD

Business Unit Director:
Susan L. Simpfenderfer

Executive Editor:
Marlene McHugh Pratt

Acquisitions Editor:
Paul Drougas

Developmental Editor:
Patricia Gillivan

Executive Production Manager:
Wendy A. Troeger

Cover Design:
Kristina Almquist

Executive Marketing Manager:
Donna J. Lewis

Channel Manager:
Wendy E. Mapstone

NOTICE TO THE READER

Publisher does not warrant or guarantee any of the products described herein or perform any independent analysis in connection with any of the product information contained herein. Publisher does not assume, and expressly disclaims, any
obligation to obtain and include information other than that provided to it by the manufacturer.

The reader is expressly warned to consider and adopt all safety precautions that might be indicated by the activities herein
and to avoid all potential hazards. By following the instructions contained herein, the reader willingly assumes all risks in
connection with such instructions.

The Publisher makes no representation or warranties of any kind, including but not limited to, the warranties of fitness
for particular purpose or merchantability, nor are any such representations implied with respect to the material set forth
herein, and the publisher takes no responsibility with respect to such material. The Publisher shall not be liable for any
special, consequential, or exemplary damages resulting, in whole or part, from the readers' use of, or reliance upon, this
material.

CONTENTS

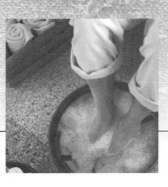

PREFACE

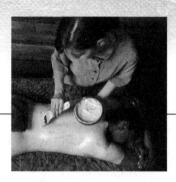

*With many traditional spa treatments being reintroduced in the United States,
The Spa Encyclopedia will serve many spa and medical professionals. It is a
much needed tool. Spa clients can also use it to inform themselves about treatments.*

*Some of the treatments described here have been around for hundreds of
years. Some of them have been scientifically or medically proven to be effective for certain ailments. Others work anecdotally, while they cannot or have
not been proven effective. After reading through The Spa Encyclopedia, one
will be familiar with the large variety of spa therapies used by clinicians,
allied health professionals, and technicians in the beauty industry. These
include the use of thermal agents, water, mechanical agents, and cosmetic
agents.*

*Research references and a glossary have been included. There is much information available in the medical literature on the effects or clinical results of the
application of heat and cold. Oftentimes, the therapist or technician will be
called upon to justify the use of a certain procedure. If he or she has carefully
reviewed the research literature beforehand, it will make providing an explanation for treatment that much easier.*

ACKNOWLEDGMENTS

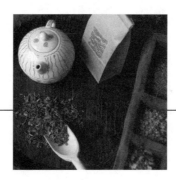

Special thanks to the following people for contributing in many ways to this book. The authors appreciate their efforts.

Catherine Atzen for her encouragement and her input on spa treatments.

Dee Deluca-Mattos for her insight in licensing.

Kelley Eubanks for her perspective from the spa consumers' point of view.

Gary M. Spolansky for his input on Reiki.

The editor(s) and staff of Delmar Learning.

Reviewers: Jane Crawford, Judith Stanton, Monica Tuma Brown, and Robin T. W. Yaun, M.D.

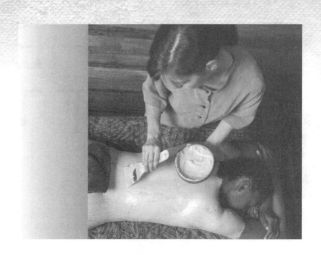

SECTION I

The World of the Spa

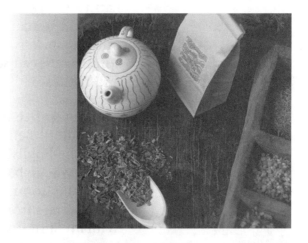

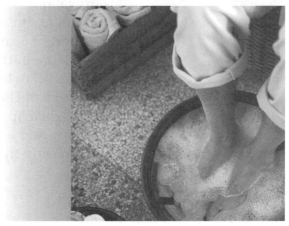

CHAPTER 1

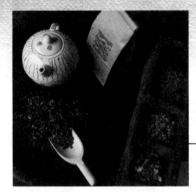

THE ORIGIN OF THE SPA

To understand how spas have developed over the last two decades in the United States, let's take a short glimpse into the history of spas. One possible source of the word *spa* is the Latin *solus per aqua,* meaning "health from water." *Spa* was (and is) the name of a small village in Belgium with hot mineral springs. The ancient Romans discovered that these springs relieved soldiers' aches and pains after long marches and battles.

Another source for the word may be the old Walloon (spoken in Southern Belgium) word for fountain, *espa.* From this came the English word *spaw* and the modern word *spa.* Again, we are back to the town of Spa, near Liege, where, in 1326, the ironmaster Collin le Loup claimed that the chalybeate waters from the local spring cured him. In 1551, William Slingsby discovered a chalybeate spring (Tewhit at Harrogate) in England with water that resembled that of Sauveniere, the spring at Spa. The discovery came to the attention of Timothy Bright, who had also tasted the waters of Sauveniere. He called the Slingsby spring the "English Spa." In 1626, Doctor Dean of York published a pamphlet on the waters of Harrogate on the advice of Bright and wrote of the "English Spaw fountain." In 1652, the French described the Harrogate waters as the "spaws" of the north. Sheridan was probably the first to call a mineral water resort a "spa."

The word *spa* is used this way only in English-speaking countries. From Germany, the term *Kurort,* meaning "place of cure," spread to eastern Europe. It has the broader implication of a health resort and, although applied primarily to watering places, could be used for a climatotherapy station as well. The German word *Bad,* as part of a geographic name, or the French equivalent *les bains,* indicates more specifically a spa, as do the Italian word *terme* and the Spanish word *baños.*

For centuries Europeans have been "taking the waters"— either soaking in them or drinking them—because of their curative elements. Physicians "prescribed the cure" to their patients to relieve rheumatism, arthritis, infertility, eye soreness, skin irritations, and more. In fact, belief in the curative powers of the baths became a whole science, and for centuries this science was taught in all major medical schools in Europe. (Even today, in most European spa towns, the "taking" of the waters is restricted, unless a consultation with, and a prescription from, the local M.D.— Kur physician—has been obtained.) Simultaneous with taking the waters or basking in radon-active caves, doctors would also prescribe treatments, such as herbal wraps, dry and wet heat treatments, massages, and more. Recommended stays for "the kur" were usually two to three weeks. Until quite recently, government health insurance in Europe covered not only the medical examinations and treatments, but also lodging and meals for two-to-three-week stays at these "Kur/cure centers." How is that for a paid vacation—and without using any vacation time or sick leave!

Traditionally, the Kur towns have a community Kur center, which acts as the official medical spa facility. It is open to all visitors to the town staying at surrounding hotels (of whom many have their own cure department and doctors), as well as the local population. Guests flock to the spa center for a day to take the Kur/cure. In addition to the medical treatments prescribed by the spa physician, visitors utilize the sauna, steam room, swimming pool, cosmetic salon, beauty salon, and masseur (all separate entities). This European practice established the first "day spa program." It was the only day spa until the American day spa began to take form.

At the turn of the twentieth century, European immigrants to the United States brought with them, among many of their customs, the spa cure concept. Spa towns started to spring up around the American continent, sponsored by local governments, states, and national parks. Unfortunately, most of them went out of business when the American Medical Association (AMA) started branding the spa cure hogwash and said its claims were only old wives' tales. Modern medical science replaced "folk wisdom" and doctors (as well as pharmaceutical companies) focused more on the treatment of disease rather than preventive practices. It became vogue to recommend taking pills instead of finding natural ways to treat the symptoms and origin of ailments. Americans opted for the fast fix.

Mineral springs spas are still in existence today in the Americas, mainly in California, Mexico, and the Pacific Northwest. The oldest operating spa town, still with its original treatment facility in the center of the city, is Berkeley Springs in West Virginia. Revival is also on the way. New York State recently invested $2 million to restore the old bathhouses in Saratoga Springs, once one of the major spa towns of the Northeast. Towns like Calistoga in California and White Sulphur Springs in West Virginia are thriving because of the mineral content of their springs.

Other forms of spas have existed in different parts of the world. The hamman, or steam baths of the Middle East, were another spa tradition, as were the Finnish sauna, the Russian bath, and the Japanese bathhouses. As a matter of fact, physicians in all of these cultures prescribed spa therapies to aid in the healing and curing of certain ailments. These treatments date to well before 0 A.D. and continue throughout the Middle Ages into the twentieth century. Even the native American Indians had spa rituals (although they, of course, did not use the word *spa* until the Europeans arrived). They even showed Ponce de Leon where he could find his Fountain of Youth!

CHAPTER 2

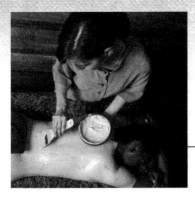

SPAS TODAY

There are a few therapeutic agents that have been used continuously for thousands of years in virtually the same form, and whose popularity has increased. Water is probably the major one of these agents. Today there are more health spas throughout the world than ever before, and more people visit them. Proponents of spa therapy may have put forth more than their share of false claims in the past—and they may continue to do so today—but there has been a fairly good balance between exaggeration and skepticism. The struggle between those for and those against will always continue, but a client with physical and/or psychological symptoms will prefer to sit out the debate in the soothing warm bath, shower, or body wrap of a health spa.

A health spa is used for therapeutic purposes. In addition to referring to a watering place, the word *spa* may also be applied to a place where the therapeutic agent is mud; or the mineral water may be in a lake or the sea. The waters may be artificial, or climate and the environment, not water, may be the principal treatment. According to some, a spa is foremost a facility where the primary interest is health.

People frequent spas for many reasons. Some seek spa treatments because scientific medicine has failed to give them the relief they crave. Others go because of the promise of relief they are told they will find or because of the relief they once did find at a spa. The word *spa* has always evoked a picture of hope. In recent years, it has come to mean a cheerful, relaxed place devoted to health. In the Europe that once was Roman, the spa visitor can see all sorts of testimonials—from ancient inscriptions to modern tablets erected by nobility. Conversely, there have always been some who say it's all in the mind, or it's all psychosomatic. Truly, it is not important whether the ailing person improves because of something physical or something psychological. What is important is that one improves.

Is there anything more to health spa therapy than psychology? Are natural mineral waters superior to reconstituted waters or synthetic preparations? Can those who insist on this prove it? Are some mineral waters superior to other mineral waters for this or that condition or patient? How is the dosage of mineral waters determined for different diseases and ailments? Is it possible that some spa regimes can affect improvement where other forms of therapy fail? Even among the experts, the range of opinions is so broad that such answers, as they may be presented, may not satisfy.

The New View of Spa Therapy

Spa physicians and therapists have begun to stress a view of spa therapy that has always existed to some degree, namely that the use of water-based spa therapies constitutes only a part of the spa regimen. While diet, exercise, stress management, hydrotherapeutic baths, and rest have always been considered inseparable components of the total prescription, today their integration is more highly empasized. Thus clinical balneotherapy (the classical treatments with mineral waters) has been undergoing a transition: from the older classical insistence on the use of natural water to the newer approach of its integration with all forms of treatments.

Although the important water at a spa is the mineral-enriched water, ordinary water has long been widely used in the form of baths, showers, irrigations, ablutions, and in other forms of balneotherapy. The swimming pool has become an increasingly important facility for exercise, and spas have developed reputations as rehabilitation and wellness centers for those with orthopedic or muscular weaknesses or syndromes.

In the United States today, there are many types of spas, to serve a variety of needs. From destination and resort spas, where the client can stay for extended periods, to day spas, where the client can go for a particular treatment or series of treatments, and from wellness centers to rehabilitation centers, there is a spa to fit every need. Let's examine the different categories of spas as they exist today in the United States.

The Destination Spa

The forerunner of the destination spa is the "fat farm." They were termed "fat farms" because they were geared toward weight loss and, sometimes, detoxification. They were where the rich and famous went to trim down, or in some cases, dry out. Many of them were run rigidly, like boot camps, with fasting and a severely restricted diet often being the core of the program. A week at such a place would achieve the promised result, but it would by no means be pleasant. Few offered relaxation or behavior modification programs, and even fewer provided beauty treatments. Because clients were not taught how to properly eat or exercise, after they left most gained back the pounds that they had lost.

Today these facilities offer delicious low-calorie foods on their menus, meaningful exercise programs (many include nature and seasonal outdoor activities), lifestyle lectures, and even medical evaluations and tests. Here every guest is a spa guest! There are no other guests around—*everyone* is there because they intend to achieve their goals, such as to lose weight, to de-stress, to build muscle tone, to eat healthy, and generally to get back on track. There are no temptations such as rich chocolate cakes or a bar. Many of these spas ban smoking on their premises (and offer smoking cessation programs) and you are expected to participate in a variety of activities—although you are not "forced" to do so. (But look, you just spent $2,500 or more for this week, why shouldn't you participate?) Note that no outside persons attend this type of spa, not even for a day.

The Resort/Hotel Spa

Many hotels and vacation resorts have added spas. The hospitality industry has seen its trends, with each hotel and resort hoping to outdo the other. The past decades have seen the swimming pool (1960s); the tennis court (1970s); the golf course and the health club (1980s); and the "spa" (1990s) is now a must, and is considered a vital part of a resort or hotel. Unlike a swimming pool, tennis court, or golf course which, once built, can't be appreciably changed, the spa lends itself to evolving services and can be adjusted to suit the changing demands of its guests.

We have to make two distinctions in the resort/hotel spa category: "amenity spas" and "resort spas."

Amenity Spa

Located at the hotel or resort, this is usually a facility that has expanded from an exercise/workout area. All services are a la carte, and facilities such as wet areas and exercise equipment are free for guests' use or available for a minimal charge. Outside guests are welcome, and many even pay a membership fee to use the amenity spa facilities regularly.

Resort Spa

This is a crossover between the resort and the destination spa. Offerings include programs similar to those at the destination spa. Many offer a separate dining room facility for spa guests. The advantage—or disadvantage—is that the temptations to get off the program/diet are very close by. Spa guests mingle with other resort guests who are there for many reasons other than spa-ing! Alcohol, smoking, high-calorie foods, and desserts are available. Determined clients can achieve the same goals at a resort spa that they would at a destination spa. If they are not determined though, they are in trouble! Many of the "all-inclusive" resorts and onboard cruise line spa programs can be counted in this category.

The Day Spa

The forerunners to the day spa were the bathhouses in metropolitan areas, salons such as the pioneer Red Door Salons of Elizabeth Arden, and, in the latter part of the twentieth century, skin care facilities such as Georgette Klinger's salons. With the popularity of destination spas growing in the late 1980s and early 1990s, skin care professionals (now called estheticians) started to offer massages and wraps, and even nutritional programs and lifestyle lectures. Thus the day spa was born, and in its present form it is purely an American invention. The whole concept is an American invention!

Today many beauty salons want to cash in on the popularity of spa treatments and have added the term *day spa* to their business names. That—forgive me—is the rub: it's perfectly fine for a gym to offer massage or a hair salon to offer a few kinds of skin treatments, but they have no more business calling themselves day spas than a first-aid station has calling itself a hospital! It is because of this trend that the Day Spa Association (DSA), a trade association, has established the following guidelines. They were established to help the spa-going public determine the difference between a day spa and a salon that offers spa services.

Essence of a Day Spa

A day spa offers:

- ❖ A clean, safe, calming, and nurturing environment.

- ❖ Private treatment rooms for each client receiving a personal service.

- ❖ Showering and changing facilities for women and men.

- ❖ Spa robes and shoes for all sizes.

- ❖ Business licenses; professional, licensed estheticians and therapists on staff.

- ❖ Professional spa products, which estheticians and therapists have been trained to use.

- ❖ Massages: Swedish, lymph drainage, and reflexology (optional: shiatsu, polarity, sports, deep tissue, and deep muscle).

- ❖ Body treatments (one or more on the menu): body packs and wraps, exfoliation, cellulite, body toning/contouring, waxing, development of home-care programs (optional: electrical impulse body toning, heat treatments, Ayurveda treatments, laser hair removal, electrolysis, hand and foot care).

- ❖ Face: cleansing facial, development of a home-care program (optional: medical facial, nonsurgical face lift, electrical toning, hair removal, electrolysis, cosmetics, make-up consultation).

- ❖ Aromatherapy: personalized for body and/or face.

- ❖ One of the following: hydrotherapy or steam and sauna.

- ❖ One of the following: nutritional counseling/weight management; private trainer/yoga/meditation; spa cuisine.

- ❖ Optional: hair—full service salon, scalp treatments, and hair packs; spa manicure and pedicure.

Club Spas

The health club industry is also jumping onto the spa bandwagon. What better place to offer spa services? Health club clients are already avid believers in healthy living and feeling good. Services offered at these facilities are for both health club members and outside customers coming in for treatments. It is best when the spa areas are far away from the bustling health club atmosphere and the facility is well insulated to keep the usual high energy and noise level of the club away from the spa atmosphere.

Medi-Spas

With the popularity of spa products and treatments reaching men and women of all ages and backgrounds, the field of esthetics has become more popular and more intricate. A cross-association with the medical industry is only natural, as the goals of beauty and wellness became synonymous. Some day spas are home to satellite offices for cosmetic surgeons and dermatologists. These associations help illustrate the correlation between spa therapies and medical treatments and help popularize the newest sector of the spa industry, the "medi-spa." Other medically oriented spas are being established nationwide by plastic surgeons, dermatologists, and chiropractors, as well as homeopathic physicians.

Wellness Centers

One-stop wellness centers are starting to be established. The concept of a wellness center is simple, convenient, and efficient: consumers can find spa and medical services all under one roof. Each service is an entity by itself, but they work together on a referral basis, with some of them having a common reception and spa/wellness coordinator. Another new concept is the longevity center, which emphasizes prolonging and improving the quality of life. This is one concept we have to watch in the next few years, as baby boomers insist on preserving their youthful appearance and living a longer, healthier life!

Rehabilitation Centers and Hospital Spas

As more and more data becomes available to the medical professions about spa treatments, progressive health care providers are starting to incorporate spa treatments into patient care. Rehabilitation centers are using such methods as Watsu (water Shiatsu), Trager massages (also called psychological integration), and Pilates (an exercise program that emphasizes flexibility and overall strength) to help their clients onto the road to recovery. Hospitals turn to spa treatments to ease the discomfort of their sick and terminally ill patients, and pain management practitioners have become firm believers in spa treatments.

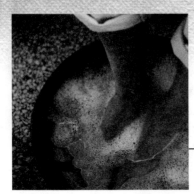

CHAPTER 3

THE SPA TREATMENTS

by Catherine Atzen

Popular Spa Treatments

Facials, peels, hair removal, body massages, and body treatments are on most spa menus. The fundamentals of the services are similar in all spas, while signature treatments, products used, and personalized methods make each spa unique. Guests select a spa for the experience, stress relief, to prevent premature aging of their skin, or to improve a condition such as acne, skin dehydration or oiliness, rosacea, psoriasis, eczema, wrinkles and loss of elasticity, dark circles or swelling of the eyes, cellulite, or heavy legs. Pre- and post-operative care reduces swelling, bruising, and discomfort.

Facials

Facials are the most popular service in spas. The facials introduced in America by European estheticians since the early 1900s have been commonly termed "European facials." They are cleansing facials, different from skin treatments. Facials take approximately an hour and include an exfoliation, a massage, steam or a warm towel application, extraction of comedones, a mask, and the application of a serum, ampoule, or essential oils. A treatment consists of the use of equipment, a specialty massage, or a mask. The esthetician educates clients on the benefits of using recommended home-care products.

Contraindications: Sores or conditions that indicate the need of medical intervention contraindicate facials. Equipment that applies electricity on the skin should not be used on guests who have a pacemaker or metal plates, or who suffer from epilepsy, diabetes, or other conditions.

Peels

The accumulation of dead skin gives skin a lifeless, ashy tone and uneven coloring. It interferes with the penetration of creams and serums into the living layers of the skin. The purpose of a peel is to slough dead skin off the epidermis. Peels unclog the hair follicles, and with regular use diminish the incidence of pustules, blackheads, and closed comedones. Post-laser resurfacing or dermabrasion, they help prevent milia and even the skin tone. They can reduce lines, wrinkles, hyperpigmentation due to sun damage or scarring, and enlarged pores. Regular peels indirectly signal the dermis cells to increase cellular activity, which makes peels an essential part of any anti-aging program.

Scrubs, also called *exfoliating grains*, are made of polypropylene, sand, or crushed seeds of apricots or other plants. The finest ones are made with very small grains to avoid irritation to the skin. Some are formulated with soothing medicinal plants, such as calendula, and are suitable for sensitive skin, acne, or for use weeks after medical peels. Scrubs get applied on wet skin with the fingertips or using a brush in a circular motion. Many scrubs are not suited for sensitive skin.

*Peeling*s are made with kaolin and white clay in a creamy substance that adheres to the skin. You can rub the peeling (which mixes with dead skin cells and impurities) off using your fingertips. Peelings are well suited for acne and oily skin.

Scrubs and peelings are used during facials, and as home-care products.

Enzyme peels are usually made of plants like papaya or pineapple. They are used as part of a facial or a treatment. These peels are in powder form, and are mixed with a toner at the time of use or dissolved in an aqueous solution. Some enzymes are formulated for all skin types and sensitive skin. The best formulations ease deep cleansing of the pores without side effects. Others may cause irritation in sensitive skin.

Alpha hydroxy acid (AHA) and chemical peels are another option. Milder AHA peels, such as glycolic acid when used in percentages ranging from 14 to 40%, get applied on the skin and then rinsed off within minutes, as part of a facial or as a separate service. They sting very little and there is no down time. The peels with low ph (2-2.5) and a high percentage of AHAs (30% and higher) work faster and deeper. The strongest AHA peels (those containing 75% glycolic acid, Jessner, or non-resorcinol peels) are even deeper peels, causing the surface of the skin to turn brown and shed within about four days. The peels are done without pain reliever. Medical supervision or access is advisable with stronger peels.

Microdermabrasion is done with equipment that projects fine inert aluminum oxide crystals, or corundum powder, through a tube to the surface of the skin. The depth of the peel depends on the setting, the power of the equipment, and the desired result. Light peels are an alternative to enzymes and AHAs. Deeper peels can improve scars, stretch marks, acne scars, and discoloration. The quality of the crystals, the equipment, the skin-care products applied, and experience all matter. There is no down time for mild peels, and the discomfort is none to mild.

Contraindications: AHAs, chemical peels, and microdermabrasion should not be administered on individuals using skin sensitizing medication, Retin A, or Accutane. Patch tests are advisable on sensitive skin.

Manual Lymph Drainage (MLD) and Lymphobiology

Manual lymph drainage (MLD) was developed by Dr. Emile Vodder in France in 1936. Dr. Vodder was seeking a therapeutic method of improving the health and quality of life of individuals suffering from fluid retention, toxicity, and various skin conditions. The method consists of a light massage that stimulates lymph circulation on the face or the body.

Lymphobiology is a proprietary science inspired by MLD; it uses equipment that produces the therapeutic massage of the manual method, but in less time, through glass tubes sliding on the skin. The equipment is classified as a therapeutic massager by the Food and Drug Administration (FDA). Information about the method has been published in medical journals following double-blind and single-blind medical studies (see "Noninvasive Techniques of Facial Rejuvenation," by Steven Bosniak, MD, and Marian Cantisano-Zilka, MD, Saunders, vol. 2, no. 4, Dec. 1999). Selected skin-care products with integral DNA are used as part of the Lymphobiology procedure to hydrate the tissues and supply nutrients at the cellular level. Lymphobiology cleanses the skin tissues of waste and toxins, and eliminates swelling and dark circles, even after only one treatment. It naturally stimulates the immune system and lowers the sympathetic nervous system, inducing deep relaxation. Redness after extractions of comedones or after peels virtually disappears. Sagging skin tightens on the face and body. The treatments can be done in series or individually; they can be added to facials, body facials, hydrotherapy, and cellulite treatments. The clinical protocol recommends treatments before and after cosmetic surgery to eliminate bruising, swelling, and discomfort, to reduce stress, to prevent cellulite from coming back after liposuction, and to improve elasticity.

Contraindications: Phlebitis. Communicate with physician before and after surgery, and when medical conditions exist. Safe to use on individuals with pacemakers or metal plates since no electricity touches the skin.

Masks

Besides the classical clay, kaolin cream, or gel masks, hydrating and clarifying treatment masks can constitute a service by themselves or be part of a facial. Specialty masks can include an ampoule, the application of a gel (usually made of algae or even single-cell algae so nutrients can penetrate), and a setting solution to turn the mask into a film that can be lifted off the skin. Masks even skin tone, eliminate redness, and tighten pores. After a mask, the skin feels like silk. Less therapeutic results are achieved with masks that are "rubbery and occlusive," or waxy such as paraffin. Clay masks harden and get removed in one dramatic-looking piece. Rubbery and hardened clay masks mainly serve cosmetic purposes, as they do not penetrate the skin with active ingredients, but just trap moisture in the stratum corneum.

Contraindications: Do not apply masks that harden on claustrophobic individuals.

Aromatherapy

Aromatherapy, or the science of using essential oils of flowers and plants for their therapeutic effect, induces healing and well-being. Essential oils can be inhaled or added to lotions during facials, treatments, and massages, and massaged into the skin.

Contraindications: Allergies, sensitivities, and wrong dosage or blend can result in rashes, nausea, headaches, and other temporary side effects.

Popular Massages and Body Treatments

Qi Gong Energy Massage

This holistic body session combines deep tissue massage to relieve muscles, ligaments, and tendons; painless pressure point Shiatsu to release energy blockages; reflexology of the feet or hands to stimulate, through the meridians, every organ; and craniosacral therapy to rebalance the individual. Qi Gong brings the body, mind, and soul into a complete state of relaxation, where all healing begins.

Myofascial Release

The fascia is a continuous elastic sheath binding together all the structures of the body. The fascia often shortens and adheres to surrounding layers of tissue, especially in the neck and back, causing tension and discomfort. Myofascial release is a deep massage involving Rolfing (named after Dr. Rolf, who researched the biochemical states of fascia) to restore elasticity and hydration to the connective tissues, and break the adhesions.

Stone Massage

Flat and smooth basal or sedimentary stones are heated in a special unit and placed on sore or tense areas in the back, in-between toes, and on different parts of the body and the face while the client lies on a massage bed. Stone therapy is very popular and has thus been expanded to include stone facials, manicures, and pedicures. Stone massage creates a relaxing and unique experience that benefits all.

Crystal Massage

Semi-precious stones are regarded as healing, and help to balance the energy of the chakra (one of the seven centers of spiritual energy in the body). Treatment with stones like tourmaline, quartz, topaz, and amethyst is often combined with stone massage, color therapy, or other massages.

Infant and Child Massage

Research demonstrates the benefits of light, calming strokes on the back, stomach, and limbs to the physical, psychological, and psychosocial well-being of babies and children. Premature babies grow faster and healthier.

Children sleep better, experience less illness, and enjoy better cognitive abilities. Massages calm anxiousness, hyperactivity, and aggressive behavior.

Pregnancy Massage

Swedish massage or accupressure can help relieve back and leg pain by improving circulation and releasing muscle tension. The client lies comfortably on her side, and avoids putting weight on the vena cava. Massage therapies such as MLD or Lymphobiology eliminate swelling, as well as fluid and waste material retention in the legs and face. This also eliminates the principal cause of cellulite.

Lipossage and Endermology

Both of these methods combine Rolfing, to detach fascia adherences, and craniosacral techniques with deep tissue massage. The manual method is meant to lengthen the spine and reduce cellulite. Endermology uses proprietary equipment claimed to be FDA-cleared to provide deep kneading massage. It was developed to break up fat deposits and improve body contours.

Back Facials and Body Facials

Following a procedure similar to that in a facial, a back facial can eliminate blackheads and dead skin cells to reveal healthy-looking skin. Regular back facials control acne and prevent scarring.

Body facials silken the skin over the body by eliminating dead skin, and dry elbows and knees. These facials use an exfoliant, peeling, loofa, glycolic peel, or salt glow.

Scalp Treatments

Therapeutic scalp treatments address itchiness, oiliness, cysts, or flakiness of the scalp; often these are related to acne on the face and back. Treating the scalp and the skin simultaneously clears acne better. Scalp treatments include relaxing massages and the application of conditioners that bring shine to the hair and health to the scalp.

Self-Tanning

A self-tanning lotion is applied on the face or body after exfoliation to achieve a tanned appearance. The client is instructed on how to maintain this look.

Follow manufacturer's instructions as some self-tanning lotions can be used as often as desired and others might be irritating if used frequently.

Nail Services

Spa manicures and pedicures are luxury versions of manicures and pedicures. They include exfoliation using scrubs, pumice stones, or glycolic acid peels, various massage methods, and the use of specialty products.

Lash and Brow Tinting, and Permanent Makeup

The hair of the lashes and brow can be tinted in a way similar to the way that hair is, using FDA-regulated formulations to prevent damage to the eyes. The color lasts for about a month. Tinting is not permitted in all states.

Permanent makeup involves applying tattoos to define eyebrows; draw eye or lip liners; or re-create the appearance of the areola after reconstructive breast surgery. Some states do not license this art. Complaints usually involve poor artistic rendering, color fading, or infections.

Hair Removal: Waxing, Laser, and Electrolysis

In *waxing*, warm wax gets applied to areas of unwanted hair, on the face, underarms, arms, bikini line, or legs. Within seconds of the wax cooling, it is pulled off using a strip of muslin (hard wax, mostly used for sensitive skin, does not require muslin). The hair grows back finer and softer after about a month. High-quality wax and following waxing with an anti-inflammatory gel will virtually eliminate sensitivity.

Laser light burns the hair at its root. After several sessions spaced over several months, this hair removal solution is permanent. Lasers do not work on dark skin as they cannot distinguish between the pigments of the skin and of the hair. Nor are lasers effective on light-colored hair since the hair lacks the pigment needed to attract the laser light.

Electrolysis uses a needle that penetrates each hair shaft directly with electrical current to permanently eliminate hair growth. The procedure is time consuming.

Contraindications: Sun exposure, use of Retin A, Accutane, AHAs, and skin sensitizing medications contraindicate these procedures. Complaints include pigmentation changes, scarring, and burns with lasers and electrolysis. The quality of equipment and skills matter. Check licensing in your state.

CHAPTER 4

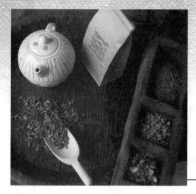

YOU, THE SPA CLIENT

How to Choose a Spa

If you have the time and the money to go away to a destination or resort spa, any of the five-day programs being offered around the United States, the Caribbean, Asia, and Europe can certainly put you on the path to healthy living. But nothing lasts forever! You must follow through on any new regime, or the effects will be lost. This is called maintenance, and this is where your local day spa comes into play. Even if you don't go the destination/resort route first, a good day spa will help you establish, and then follow, a healthful regime.

You must first decide what you want to achieve, and then find the right spa. The color insert in this book is a directory of day spas that have joined the Day Spa Association (DSA) and that take their calling seriously. The DSA offers an accreditation to day spas that have met the guidelines listed in Chapter 2. Many of the spas listed have been accredited by the DSA; others, although meeting the guidelines, have not yet applied for their accreditation status, but are highly recommended as bona-fide and licensed day spa businesses.

First of all, let's start with what you want to achieve.

❖ Is it beautiful skin? Then make sure the spa you choose offers at least three types of skin care products so that they can advise you which one would be best for your skin type.

❖ Is it relief from an aching body or tight muscles? Then make sure the spa you choose offers various types of massages that can be applied to your particular problem.

❖ Is it detoxification or easing water retention and bloating? Then make sure the spa you choose offers lymphatic treatments and body/herbal wraps.

❖ Is it just relaxation? Make sure the spa you choose has some of the water treatments known to calm nerves and let you forget gravity.

❖ Is it weight loss or exercise? Make sure the spa you choose has a nutritionist and private trainer on staff, or is aligned with a health club.

Spa Licensing and Personnel Training

Whatever spa you choose, be sure the most basic licensing is in place.

1. **Licensed establishments:** Each state has its own licensing requirements. In most states, each technician as well as the facility must be licensed. Depending on the state, the licenses may be issued by the board of cosmetology or the board of health. Check to be sure that the appropriate licensing is in place.

2. **Licensed esthetician:** An esthetician undergoes practical and hands-on training regarding the skin and has to be licensed by the local cosmetology board. License requirements vary from state to state. Some states will allow estheticians to work only on your face and neck, others will allow body work and more intricate treatments. An esthetician also needs to be trained on the application of each specialized skin care product. Make sure that the person working on you, using a certain product, can produce proof that she or he has taken the proper manufacturer's training classes.

3. **Licensed massage therapist:** A massage therapist undergoes extensive training regarding the body, muscles, and tissues, and a multitude of massage techniques on the body. Once licensed, a therapist must attend a predetermined number of postgraduate training classes to retain his or her license. The license is granted by their state massage therapy board. Again, the requirements vary greatly from state to state.

4. **Certified massage therapist:** A certified massage therapist undergoes training in massage therapy techniques. Although trained in massage, he or she doe not undergo the intense training that a licensed therapist does.

5. **Spa therapist:** A spa therapist is usually licensed in massage and esthetics and is cross-trained to administer specific spa treatments such as hydrotherapy (water treatments), aromatherapy, wraps, and baths. A spa therapist must have proper training in the operation of the particular apparatus he or she is using, as well as a thorough knowledge of the body's anatomy. Some treatments, when performed by nonprofessionals, can do you more harm than good. There are spa therapy training institutes in the United States and educational courses available that issue certificates; look for them displayed prominently in the treatment areas of the spa. There is no formal licensing available as of yet for this type of therapist. **Note:** Some states insist that some spa treatments be performed only under the supervision of a physician. Make sure you know the "law of the land."

6. **The staff:** Ask about the staff's training programs. There are new treatments and products coming onto the market daily. Spa owners and managers need to have a continuous education program in place for their personnel.

7. **The spa itself:** Last but not least, look for cleanliness. In today's age, with so many diseases, this is the most obvious factor of all. Insist that sterilized accessories are used on your skin, and that the therapists wear gloves at all times. Fresh linen and towels must be the norm.

Signature Treatments

What are "signature treatments"? Spas are trying to outdo each other, to distinguish themselves from each other. Many create special treatments using the natural resources from the area in which they are located. We heard how the mineral contents of certain springs can help cure certain ailments (e.g., sulphur is an excellent healing source for rheumatism, the Dead Sea carries minerals that help with psoriasis, moor peat packs help inflammation of the nervous system, and so on). There are also myths, such as of springs that will help men become more productive or help relieve or cure female reproductive illnesses.

Stories are told that in the eighteenth and nineteenth centuries, emperors and kings would take the baths at various spa towns in order to produce an heir. It happened, but not necessarily because of the waters. It could have been due to their state of relaxation, or maybe a new liaison they started while at the spa?

In any case, be sure to ask exactly what these signature treatments will accomplish. Some of them are designed to awaken your interest or to help you choose a certain spa over another, and some are just pure advertising gimmicks that will have little therapeutic effects. A chocolate- or strawberry-flavored wrap may be the answer to your prayers, but it certainly will not achieve any more than a plain wrap—and definitely *less* than an herbal wrap!

Your Expectations

What should you expect from a spa? You have the right to know!

❖ Spa personnel should be courteous and friendly.

❖ The spa staff should inquire about any allergies or health conditions of which they should be aware. If they do not inquire, you should volunteer this information.

❖ You should be offered a brief explanation of the treatment that is being or will be administered.

❖ Answers should be provided to any questions you may have about your treatment, the products used, maintaining results, and so on.

❖ A quiet space for relaxing should be available between services, a place where you will not feel exposed or embarrassed.

❖ You should receive your full treatment time, unless you are late.

❖ Prompt resolution to any problem that arises with your treatment should be offered.

❖ Spa policies should be available and discussed at the time of booking (e.g., some spas charge one-half or the entire treatment cost when a cancellation occurs within less than twenty-four hours of the appointment).

❖ A technician of the same gender should be available if you are uncomfortable with one of the opposite sex providing treatment.

❖ You have the right to be draped/covered at all times, with only the area of your body that is being worked exposed to the therapist (and the world!).

Your Responsibilities

As a client, you also have responsibilities to the spa. You need to make sure you live up to your end of the bargain!

❖ Before you book a spa stay, be sure you know as much as possible about the program(s) and treatment(s). Ask, ask, ask, and learn as much as you can.

❖ If you decide to go away for a spa retreat, make sure the spa is right for you. If you'd like to lose a few pounds and expect to go on a diet, you should choose a spa that offers this. Don't expect a diet menu at a spa that is strictly a beauty/pampering facility.

❖ Be careful when choosing your spa. If you don't care for yoga and meditation, then don't choose a get-away that is known for getting you up at 5:00 A.M. to meditate on the beach when the sun rises! If hiking is what you are looking for, you should choose a spa whose fitness program is not aerobic classes and the treadmill, but a morning hike in the mountains, the desert, or on a country road.

❖ If you want pampering at a day spa, then be sure the treatments you book are just that. If you want to achieve firming, body contouring, inch loss, or water loss, then you need to book the appropriate treatment at a day spa that offers these. That doesn't mean you can't be pampered, too!

Spa Etiquette

1. Be on time for your appointment. Arriving half an hour earlier will allow you to get in the right frame of mind and will allow the spa staff to get ready for you.

2. If you come from home, leave your jewelry, pocketbook, unnecessary monies, and credit cards at home. If you come from work, or need these accessories for going out after your spa visit, make sure you lock them up in the spa's safe. Time and time again (it happened to the

writer, too!) we put our ring or watch into the pocket of the bathrobe provided by the spa and then forget about it. The staff does sometimes forget to check the pockets, and your watch winds up in the laundry—which is often done outside the premises by a third party. There is no one to blame but yourself! (Now if you encounter a spa that gives you a bathrobe without pockets, you'll know why!)

3. Allow plenty of time for relaxation after your treatments. In order to derive the most benefit from your spa visit, take time to linger after the kneading, poking, squeezing, sweating, and soaking (depending on what you are having done) is over. You owe it to yourself to let the experience and the therapeutic effect sink into you and recharge your energies. Rushing off to your next appointment without proper rest will only cancel out what you just tried to do!

4. Be courteous toward the staff. We are all human, and we all have good days and bad days. The spa staff is trained to be nurturing and caring and patient. Complaints about a therapist or anything you do not like should be made to management only, and should be objective and done in a professional manner.

5. Be honest in filling out the medical evaluation sheet. This will help the spa staff watch out for any contraindications a certain treatment or product may have for your condition or on your skin.

6. Ask questions of the therapist. Insist that she or he explains to you what is being done, what kind of products are being used, and their effect on you.

7. Tipping is usually not included in the price of your treatment at day spas. You are expected to leave a tip of at least 10 percent of the treatment price. Many spas have envelopes at the front desk in which you can leave your gratuities—a separate one for each therapist. Check with the front desk manager before you start your spa visit about the policy, so you are prepared to act appropriately. Many destination/resort spas will include gratuities (usually 15 percent) in the overall bill for your spa stay—covering tipping for treatments, dining room, and other services. Tipping at these facilities is most often not required or necessary; however, it is always a good idea to check with the reservation agent. Policies are usually also spelled out clearly in a spa's brochure.

8. In order to reach the goals you set out to achieve, be sure to follow your therapists' instructions completely. When purchasing a home-care regime, insist that it be written out for you. Although you may

think that you will remember it all, not too many people do when they get home! Just as your family physician and your pharmacist give you detailed instructions about the medicine you take, you should accept the same careful approach to the instructions given by the spa. Remember, spa therapists are professionals who have studied hard (and are always continuing to learn more). They are the experts in their field. After all, that is why you are buying your treatment products from them, and not from the cosmetic counter of your department store!

9. Buy the treatment series. It will save you money and will assure that you follow through with your intention. It will help you achieve the results you set out to get!

If you follow these suggestions, your spa visit will definitely give you the results you desire, and assure you a hassle-free, safe, and enjoyable time. Please do remember that spa therapists are people, too—they are by nature nurturing individuals who are not only trained in the treatments they give and products they use, but they are transferring their positive energy to you, the client, through the magic power of touch— and a smile!

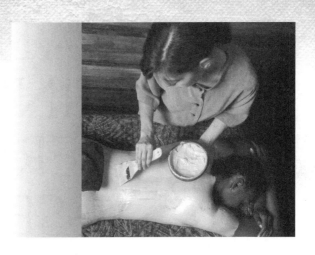

SECTION II
The Treatments

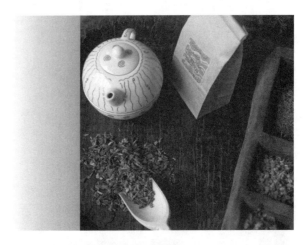

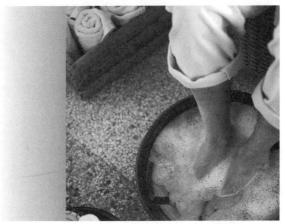

CHAPTER 5

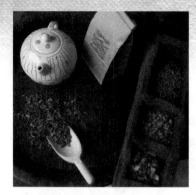

WATER, MINERAL, HERBAL, AND ESSENTIAL OIL BATH THERAPIES

Neutral Bath

BATH TREATMENTS

Definition:	The neutral bath, sometimes called the *continuous bath*, is a non-thermic hydrotherapy of great value. It consists of whole body immersion in water approximately 92 to 97°F.
Indications:	Insomnia, nervous exhaustion, anxiety, depression
Contraindications:	Diabetes, arteriosclerosis, fever, acute hypertension, chronic pain, toxemia of pregnancy, peripheral edema, cardiac weakness, eczema or other skin condition aggravated by water
Equipment:	Full-size bathtub, bath thermometer, towels, pillow, sheet
Procedure:	Fill full-size bathtub with water of neutral temperature.
	Make client comfortable with pillow or rolled towel for neck support; adjust water to temperature neutral to client. Client should feel somewhere between "comfortably warm" and neither warm nor cold. This is a better guide than the thermometer, although the actual temperature also should be monitored.
	Cover any exposed parts (e.g., knees), with towels, or cover whole tub with sheet.
	Lighting should be dim.
	Add water, as necessary, to maintain neutral temperature.
	Cool water a few degrees at the end of the treatment and assist client out of tub.

Dry quickly but gently without friction, which would be too stimulating for a calmative treatment.

Let client rest for half an hour.

Duration: Fifteen minutes to one hour for insomnia

BATH TREATMENTS

Hot Bath

Definition: The hot bath treatment consists of full immersion in water approximately 104°F. The entire body, with the exception of the head, is immersed in water. While immersed, the body cannot control its temperature by sweating; although the client's body can release some heat through the head. The body temperature rises and the detoxification process begins.

Indications: Poor circulation, pain, muscle stiffness and general fatigue, congestion of internal organs

Contraindications: Heart disease; diabetes; diseases of malignant origin such as acute cancer, acute swelling, and wounds; vascular disorders; high blood pressure

Procedure: Fill tub two-thirds full of hot water. The temperature should be 104°F. Assist client into tub.

Cover exposed body parts with a towel or cover tub with a sheet or light blanket.

Keep head cool with a cold compress.

Check pulse regularly. Do not let pulse exceed eighty beats per minute.

Assist client from tub.

Follow the bath with an alcohol rub or a cool sponge bath.

Dry thoroughly and keep client warm.

Let client rest one hour after treatment.

Duration: One to twenty minutes

> ### WARNING
>
> Frail people will not tolerate hot bath well. If dizziness or faintness develops, stop at once. Never leave the client alone.

Cold Bath

Definition: The cold tub bath is a powerful stimulant. Use only with well conditioned clients. Treatment consists of full immersion in water approximately 75°F.

Indications: Gradual vascular conditioning, common cold in an otherwise healthy person, following a strong heat treatment, fever

Contraindications: Weakness from an infection, cardiac disease, chilliness (heat first), menstruation, allergy to cold, severe diabetes

Procedure: Fill the tub two-thirds full with water. The temperature should be about 75°F.

Assist client into tub.

Rub client vigorously with bath mitten.

Assist client from tub.

Dry client thoroughly.

Duration: Five seconds

BATH TREATMENTS

Whirlpool Bath

Definition: The whirlpool bath combines the thermal stimulus of the water with further mechanical stimuli. One way in which this occurs is with the aid of a rotating propeller, which moves the water. In addition, warm air is injected into the water through a small nozzle. Depending on its size, the whirlpool bath can be used either as a partial bath for the lower legs or the arms,

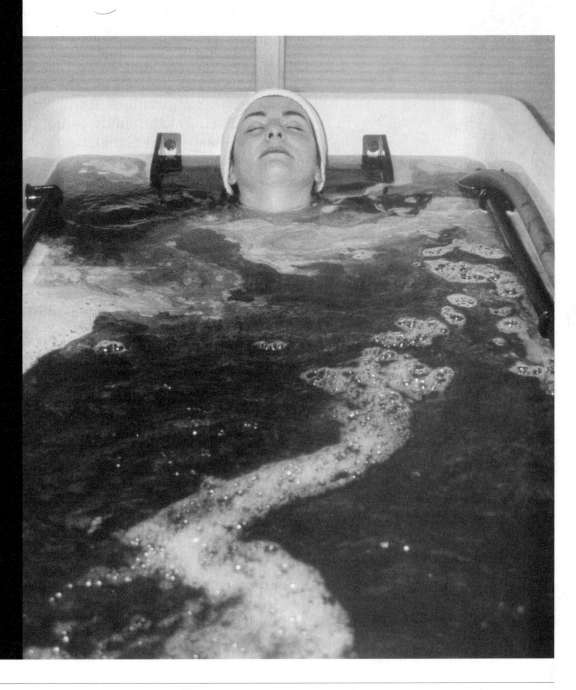

or as a full bath for the entire body. The whirlpool bath should not be compared to the underwater massage, as the mechanical component is weaker. One of the outstanding therapeutic uses of the whirlpool is to relieve muscle soreness and fatigue. This is the reason many athletes and dancers purchase portable whirlpools for their baths, or go swimming in a pool with such whirlpool action. Whirlpool baths are helpful in anti-pain therapy.

Indications: Injuries, rheumatic disabilities, including rheumatic muscle and joint disorders, muscle soreness, fatigue, Raynaud's disease, tennis elbow, knee joint problems, swollen joints of arthritis, to improve the circulation of paraplegic and polio victims. Whirlpool therapy can help with circulation problems and it is a well-known aid in relieving chronic pain and the phantom pain that occurs after amputations. It will also help to heal skin sores and infected wounds, reduce the swelling of chronic edema (tissue swelling), help reduce the pain of minor frostbite, ease scar tissue from burns, and help with weak and painful feet. Many physiotherapists prepare their clients for therapy massage by first giving them a stimulating and relaxing whirlpool bath.

Contraindications: Sensitive to very hot water, diabetes, varicose veins, advanced arteriosclerosis, or any advanced vascular limb problem

Procedure: Assist client into tub.

Start the whirlpool bath at a neutral temperature, and raise to the tolerance of the client.

Allow client to relax in tub.

Assist client from tub. If you are following the whirlpool with a massage, wrap the entire body so that it stays completely warm.

Duration: Fifteen to forty-five minutes, depending on the purpose for which it is being used

The Kneipp Baths

In the Kneipp treatments, baths are given as:

❖ Arm bath

❖ Foot bath

❖ Hip bath

❖ Half bath

❖ Three-quarter bath

❖ Full bath

These baths may be taken (temperature):

❖ Cold   32–65°F

❖ Cool   66–71°F

❖ Lukewarm   72–82°F

❖ Intermediate   83–95°F

❖ Warm   96–100°F

❖ Hot   101–105°F

Warm baths may be taken with herbal additives such as balm mint, chamomile, lavender, meadow flower, or pine needle.

The strength of the stimulus is determined by:

❖ Temperature

❖ Location and size of area

❖ Length of application

❖ Individual pretreatment disposition

BATH TREATMENTS

Arm Bath–Cold Temperature

Indications:	Fatigue, heart palpitations, tennis elbow, physical exhaustion
Contraindications:	Angina pectoris, heart ailments, cold hands
Effects:	Lowers heart rate, refreshes, decreases hypertension
Equipment:	Comfortable chair, arm bath or wash basin
Procedure:	Place client in comfortable chair.
	Fill the arm bath with cold water, 37 to 65°F.
	Dip both arms into the water, to the middle of the upper arm.
	Wipe off arms with hands.
	Do not towel dry.
	Arm exercises or bed rest should follow the arm bath. The arms should be kept warm.
Duration:	Thirty seconds (depends on water temperature), or until it is too uncomfortable. Best performed in the early afternoon.

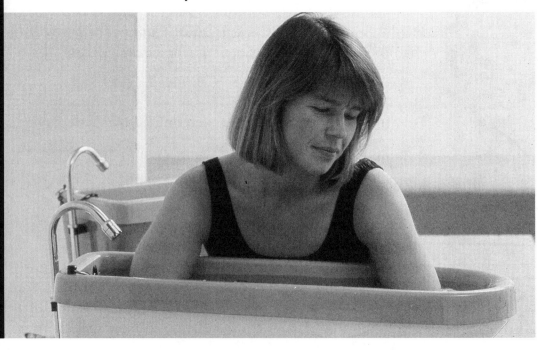

Arm Bath—Warm Temperature

Indications:	Local non-inflammatory rheumatism, arthritis of the hand, angina pectoris, bronchitis, chronic cold hands
Contraindications:	Lymph blockage, lymph edema, high blood pressure, heart ailments
Effects:	Expands mobility, antispasmodic, soothes, opens bronchi
Equipment:	Comfortable chair, arm bath or wash basin
Procedure:	Place client in comfortable chair.
	Fill the arm bath with warm water, 96 to 100°F.
	Dip both arms in the arm bath, to the middle of the upper arm.
	Towel dry arms. Let client rest at least twenty to thirty minutes.
Duration:	Fifteen to twenty minutes
Herbal Bath Additives:	Balm mint, chamomile, lavender, meadow flower, pine needle, rosemary

BATH TREATMENTS

Arm Bath—
Alternate Temperature

Indications: Blood circulation problems, high blood pressure, bronchitis

Contraindications: Angina pectoris, heart ailments

Effects: Increases blood circulation

Equipment: Comfortable chair, two arm baths or was basins

Procedure: Have client seated comfortably.

Fill one arm bath with warm water, 96 to 100°F.

Fill another arm bath with cold water, 65°F.

Dip both arms in the warm water, up to the middle of the upper arm.

Repeat the procedure in cold water.

Wipe off the arms with hands. Do not towel dry.

Exercise arms until warm.

One hour of bed rest is recommended.

Duration:
1. Five minutes warm water
2. Ten seconds cold water
3. Five minutes warm water
4. Ten seconds cold water

Herbal Bath Additives:
In warm water only: Balm mint, chamomile, lavender, meadow flower, pine needle, rosemary

Arm Bath—
Increasing Temperature

Indications:	Angina pectoris, high blood pressure, cardiovascular insufficiency, headache, asthma, bronchitis, local non-inflammatory rheumatism
Contraindications:	Lymph blockage, lymph edema of the arms, varicose veins
Effects:	Vasodilatation, improves blood circulation
Equipment:	Comfortable chair, arm bath or wash basin
Procedure:	Have client seated comfortably.
	Fill the arm bath with warm water, 83 to 95°F.
	Dip both arms in arm bath, up to middle of upper arm.
	Raise the temperature of water gradually to 105°F. (This should take fifteen to twenty minutes).
	Towel dry arms, fifteen to thirty minutes.
	Bed rest is recommended.
Duration:	Fifteen to twenty minutes
Herbal Bath Additives:	Balm mint, chamomile, lavender, meadow flower, pine needle, rosemary

Foot Bath–Cold Temperature

Indications: Venous circulatory disorders, tired feet

Contraindications: Acute bladder/kidney infections, oversensitivity to cold, female pelvic disorders, coronary deficiencies

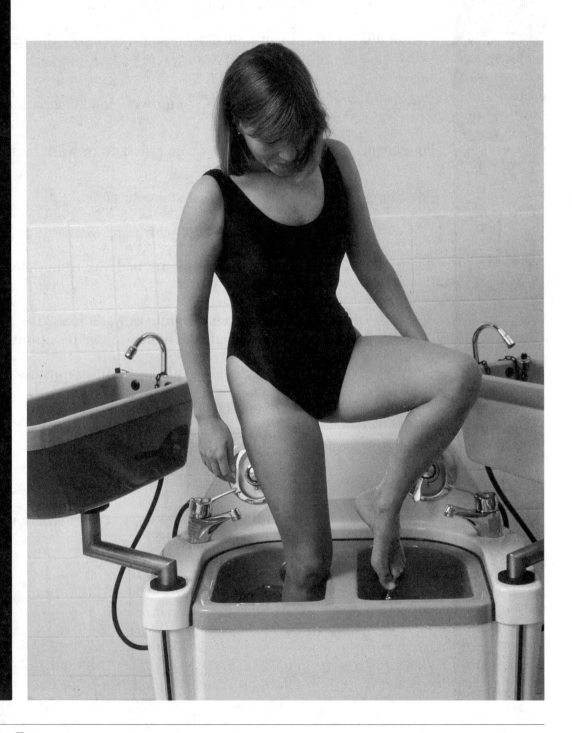

Effects: Stimulates metabolism, alleviates insomnia, sleep inducing in the evening, influences venous blood flow return, increases blood circulation

Equipment: Foot bathtub or large bucket

Procedure: Fill the footbath with cold water, 54°F.

With the water as cold as client can tolerate, instruct client to dip both feet into footbath. The client can sit in a chair or stand for this procedure, whichever is most comfortable.

Wipe water off feet with hands. Do not towel dry.

To keep feet warm, leg exercises or bed rest should follow the treatment.

Duration: Fifteen seconds to one minute

Foot Bath—Warm Temperature

Indications: Arterial circulation disorders, chronic infection (e.g.,
nose, throat, pharyngeal), weak immune system,
chronic constipation, chronic cold feet, preparation
for pedicure, after acute phase of ankle/foot contusion

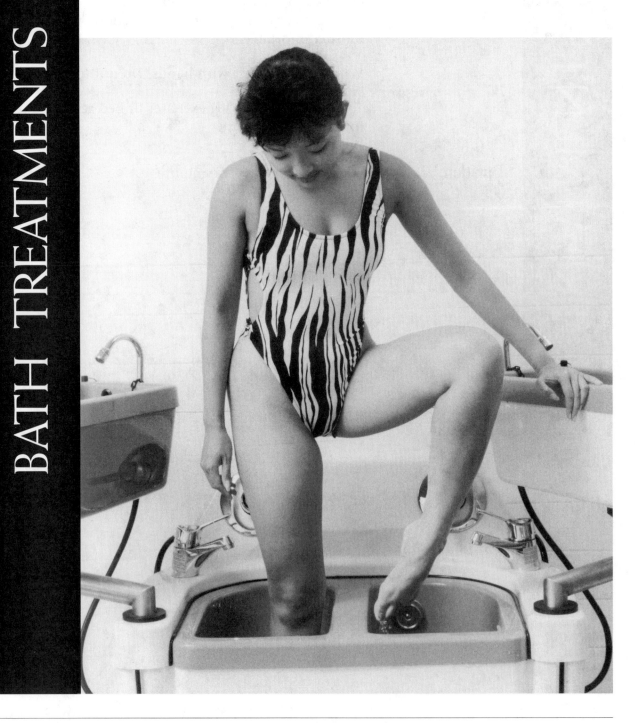

BATH TREATMENTS

Contraindications:	Varicose veins, hypertension
Effects:	Increases blood circulation, alleviates insomnia, soothes, relaxes
Equipment:	Foot bathtub or large bucket
Procedure:	Fill the footbath with warm water, 97 to 100°F.
	Instruct the client to dip both feet in the water.
	Towel dry feet.
	Follow with bed rest for at least thirty minutes.
Duration:	Ten to fifteen minutes
Herbal Bath Additives:	Balm mint, chamomile, lavender, meadow flower, pine needle, rosemary

Foot Bath—
Alternate Temperature

Indications: Chronic cold feet, low blood pressure, insomnia

Contraindications: Varicose veins

Effects: Increases effectiveness of the body's heat regulatory system, improves blood circulation, stabilizes the nervous system

Equipment: Two foot bathtubs or two large buckets

Procedure: Fill one bath with warm water, 97 to 100°F, and one bath with cold water, as cold as the client can tolerate.

Instruct the client to put both feet in the warm water for five minutes, then into the cold water for ten to fifteen seconds.

Repeat the procedure.

Wipe feet with hands. Do not towel dry.

Exercise legs until warm or follow with bed rest for one hour.

Duration: 1. Five minutes warm water

2. Ten to fifteen seconds cold water

3. Five minutes warm water

4. Ten to fifteen seconds cold water

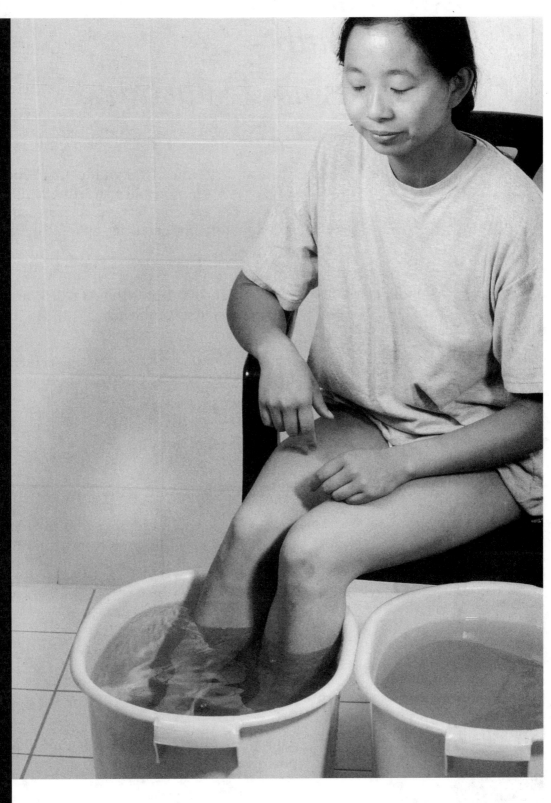

BATH TREATMENTS

Herbal Bath Additives: For warm water only: Balm mint, chamomile, lavender, meadow flower, pine needle, rosemary

Foot Bath–
Increasing Temperature

Indications: Acute and chronic bladder/kidney infections, beginning colds (symptoms like sneezing, chills, feeling weak and tired), cold feet, vascular headache, non-inflammatory problems, leg cramps, menstrual problems

Contraindications: Varicose veins, phlebitis (blood clots), heart problems, minor circulatory problems

Effects: Increases blood circulation to organs (i.e., pelvic areas). Increases body temperature in feet immediately.

Equipment: Foot bathtub or large bucket

Procedure: Fill the foot bath with warm water 83 to 95°F.

Gradually raise water temperature to 101 to 103°F. (This should take fifteen to twenty minutes.)

Towel dry feet.

Follow with bed rest for at least fifteen to thirty minutes.

Duration: Fifteen to twenty minutes

Herbal Bath Additives: Balm mint, chamomile, lavender, meadow flower, pine needle, and rosemary

Mineral, Herbal, and Essential Oil Baths

There are many herbal and pharmaceutical substances that can be added to baths to produce special effects.

Water by itself has a remarkable, almost magical ability to alter the body state. Depending on the specific need, water will decrease or increase muscle tone, reduce pain, or generate energy. The addition of certain herbal and pharmaceutical substances to the water is a twin present to the body. Some herbs soothe, others sedate or stimulate, and others soften the skin. Most important is the ability of some substances to hasten perspiration or to stimulate release of stored toxins from within the body. This ability helps to overcome many symptoms, and can improve a chronic condition.

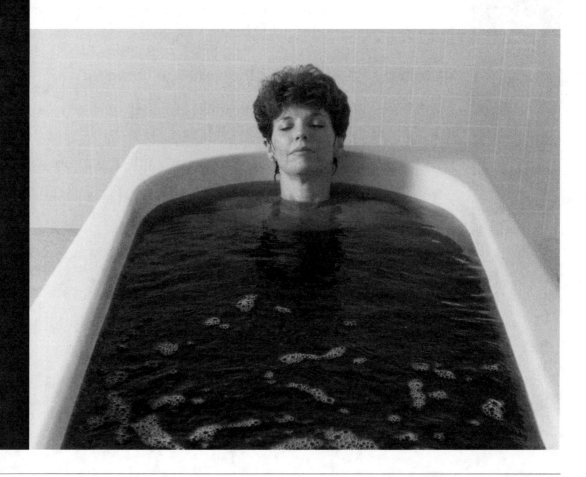

Fango (Mud) Salicyl Powder Bath

Definition: This bath is the ultimate. It is the favorite fragrant mud bath in European spa Kur therapy centers. Its soothing effects are due to the combination of the analgesic properties of the volcanic ash powder (fango) and the pine needle essential oil.

Indications: Rheumatism in muscles and joints, sciatica, neuritis, degenerative non-inflammatory joint arthrosis, lumbago

Effects: Stimulates circulation, replaces minerals, exfoliates the skin

Equipment: Bathtub, shower, towels, fango (mud) salicyl powder (ingredients: salicyl powder, natrium humat, pine needle extract)

Procedure: Dissolve the powder in hot water.

Assist client into bath, and allow to soak for ten to twenty minutes.

Assist client from bath and into a cool shower.

Wrap client in warm blanket and allow to rest.

Whey Powder Bath

BATH TREATMENTS

Definition:

Whey is a high-protein milk serum. Liquid cow's milk has about 6.25 percent protein; of that, 80 percent is contained in the whey. Traditionally, the term *whey protein* describes those milk proteins that remain after the cheese-making process uses up the casein molecules. In bygone days, whey was fed to young livestock on the farm because of its nutritional value.

Whey is a complete protein containing all the essential and non-essential amino acids found in nature. Long ago Hippocrates promoted the health and beauty benefits of whey. It was also very popular during the Renaissance. Today it is Europe's foremost skin care bath product.

It is also called "lacto-med-derm bath" (*lacto* meaning produced from milk, *med* meaning medically tested, and *derm* for skin friendly).

Indications:

Particularly useful for aging and dry skin, neurodermatitis, psoriasis, acne, eczema, baby rash, fungus, sunburn, and other skin ailments

Equipment:

Bathtub, towel, washcloth, whey bath powder (ingredients: lactose, milk fat, milk protein, graham salt, magnesium carbonate, wintergreen essential oil)

Procedure for bath:

Client should be encouraged to bathe in the whey bath at least three times per week.

Fill tub two-thirds full with warm water, 95°F.

Assist client into bath.

Allow client to soak ten to twenty minutes.

Procedure for mask:

The whey powder can also be used as a mask on the face, hands, and feet.

Assure client's comfort.

Apply powder to a wet, warm washcloth.

Apply washcloth to client's skin (face, hands, and/or feet).

Remove after ten to fifteen minutes.

BATH TREATMENTS

Mud Natrium Powder Bath

Definition: The fango (mud) natrium powder bath, used in spas worldwide, is a mineral-rich volcanic ash extract. This ancient beauty ritual is effective for removing impurities and smoothing the texture of the skin so it can readily absorb moisture and minerals.

Fango (mud) natrium powder is biologically pure, bacteria free, unscented, and fully dissolves in bath water. It will not stain the tub or body.

Indications: Tired muscles

Effects: Will detoxify and revitalize the body

Equipment: Bathtub, shower, towels, fango (mud) natrium powder (ingredients: 100% unscented natrium humat volcanic ash extract)

Procedure: Fill bathtub two-thirds full.

Dissolve powder into bath.

Assist client into tub, and allow to soak for ten to twenty minutes.

For a real spa Kur treatment, let the client shower with cool or cold water after the bath.

Client should then rest, while warmly wrapped, for ten to twenty minutes.

Mustard Powder Bath

BATH TREATMENTS

Definition: The great healing virtues of mustard have been extolled by numerous civilizations for thousands of years. The Greeks, including Hippocrates, the Romans, the early American settlers, and Native Americans all used mustard for medicinal purposes. The most universally known use of mustard is in a mustard plaster, recommended for common congestions of the lung.

Traditionally, mustard is renowned for its stimulating, cleansing, and rejuvenating qualities. The warmth of the mustard assists in opening pores, helping the body to sweat out impurities. The powder can be blended with essential oils of wintergreen (antiseptic astringent), eucalyptus (antiseptic balsamic, cooling), rosemary (calming, soothing skin tonic), and thyme (antiseptic, stimulant). These natural oils leave your skin feeling soothed and refreshed.

Indications: Fatigue, muscle and joint soreness, insomnia

Equipment: Bathtub, shower, towels, mustard powder (ingredients: powdered mustard seed, essential oils of wintergreen, eucalyptus, rosemary, thyme, sodium carbonate)

Procedure: Fill a tub two-thirds full with warm-hot water.

Dissolve two large tablespoons of the powder into the bath.

Assist client into bath, where he or she should soak for fifteen to twenty minutes.

Assist client out of the bath, and into a cool shower. Keep the shower brief.

Allow client to rest, wrapped in a warm blanket.

Seaweed Powder Bath

BATH TREATMENTS

Definition: Deep freezing and drying the seaweed (by lyophilization) conserves the product's natural qualities in a way no other method can. It conserves mineral salts, vitamins, enzymes, and the aroma.

Effects: Stimulates blood circulation, helps eliminate toxins, aids in toning the skin, restores mineral salts and trace elements

Equipment: Bathtub, shower, towels, seaweed powder

Procedure: Prepare the bath by adding two ounces of seaweed powder to 40 to 50 gallons (150–200 liters) of warm water, 102°F.

Assist client into bath, and ensure his or her comfort.

Place a cool damp towel on client's forehead.

Allow client to relax in the bath for fifteen to twenty minutes, or longer, if client is comfortable. Check on the client every ten minutes.

Provide client with plenty of liquid to drink.

A subsequent half-hour rest, with client wrapped in a warm bathrobe or blanket, will increase effectiveness of bath. The rest period prolongs perspiration and the consequent elimination of toxins.

Follow with as cold a shower as possible.

Herbal Essential Oil Baths

Definition: Herbal bath oils are highly concentrated extracts that contain vitamins, hormones, antibiotics, and antiseptics. In a warm bath the oils are absorbed through the skin, inducing deep relaxation that reduces stress, tension, and muscle aches.

Equipment: Bathtub, towels, herbal essential oils

Procedure: Prepare bath by adding two ounces of herbal oil to 40 to 50 gallons (150–200 liters) of warm water, 102°F.

Assist client into bath, and ensure his or her comfort.

Place a cool, damp towel on client's forehead.

Let client relax in tub for fifteen to twenty minutes, or longer if client is comfortable. Check on the client every ten minutes.

Provide client with plenty of liquid to drink.

BATH TREATMENTS

Bicarbonated Bath

Definition: Bicarbonated minerals are effervescent salts. When added to warm bath water, they create an effervescent bath. They ease minor aches and pains, and detoxify the skin.

Indications: Stress, minor pain, minor dermatological problems, high blood pressure, vegotonic and respiratory conditions, muscle fatigue

Equipment: Bathtub, shower, towels, bicarbonate salts (ingredients: natrium hydrogen carbonate and aluminum sulphate)

Procedure: Fill bathtub two-thirds full with warm water, 86° to 98°F.

Add bag one of bicarbonate—15 ounces (429 grams) of natrium hydrogen carbonate.

Assist client into bath water.

Add bag two of bicarbonate—18 ounces (508 grams) of aluminum sulphate pebbles.

The bicarbonate development will begin.

Let client bathe for twenty minutes, or until all pebbles are dissolved.

Follow bath with a cool or cold shower.

Let client rest, warmly wrapped, for thirty minutes.

Oxygen Bath

Definition: The oxygen-activated bath salts develop smooth pearl bubbles across the skin. They are very soothing, and help release tension, increase physical vitality, regenerate the nervous and metabolic systems, and improve blood circulation in arms and legs.

Equipment: Bathtub, shower, towels, oxygen salts (ingredients: natriumporcarbonate with 13.5% active oxygen)

Procedure: Dissolve the content of the salt, which is the oxygen carrier, in 97°F bath water.

Assist client into the bath.

Add the oxygen activator. Pearl-like oxygen bubbles will begin to form and cover the skin.

Allow client to relax in bath for twenty minutes.

Assist client out of bath, and into a cool shower.

Follow with rest, with client warmly wrapped, for one hour.

CHAPTER 6

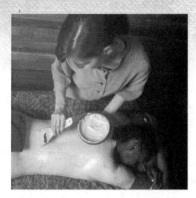

MASSAGE, WELLNESS, AND PHYSIOTHERAPIES

Massage

The physiological effects of classic massage are primarily due to its influence on muscle tone. Muscles and connective tissues are better able to withstand loosening and stretching exercises after a massage. Research has shown that constriction of the capillaries in a muscle causes a decrease in metabolism and a corresponding high degree of conduction loss and cell degeneration. Massage regulates muscle tone by enhancing circulation and localized metabolic rates. It also increases the flexibility of the muscle.

An effect on the subcutaneous (under the skin) fat layer and connective tissues, together with increased circulation in the muscles and skin, can be observed after a massage. Scientific findings concerning the effects of massage include the more rapid removal of metabolic wastes, the removal of old adhesions, and the effect of reflex massage techniques at peripheral sites, as well as the reactive effects on the vascular system and the entire body.

One of the most persistent false impressions held by both medical personnel and laypersons is the belief that massage is capable of increasing strength. Strengthening, in the physi-

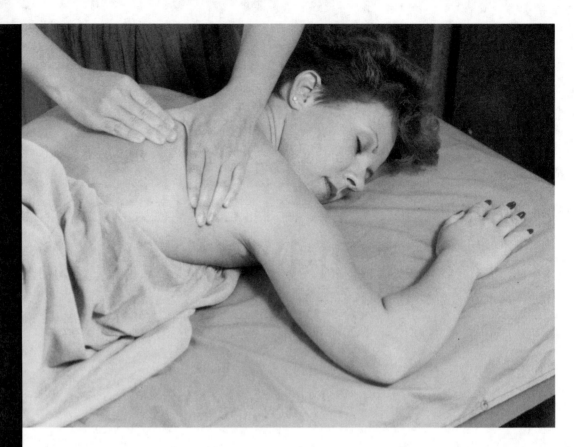

ological sense, is possible solely through targeted active exercise and systematic training. This is true both for the muscular system and the cardiovascular system. However, a massage can prepare the body for strengthening exercises by promoting the removal of waste materials in muscles and connective tissue. Moreover, massage can have a positive effect on the human psyche. It promotes relaxation, calm, and a general sense of wellbeing, if performed correctly.

During the course of a therapy program, a client will probably experience one or more of the techniques described below. Among these special massage techniques are: shiatsu, Swedish massage, reflexology, deep fascia manipulation, underwater pressure massage, and athletic massage.

Shiatsu

Shiatsu is a traditional Japanese massage technique. It was developed from ancient Chinese acupressure, which is based on energy flow through pathways in the body (meridians). These meridians, or energy pathways, are usually divided into six passive and six active groups. The six primary passive and active meridian groups are related to particular organs and to an interactive energy flow.

Shiatsu uses hand manipulation to exert pressure, ranging from gentle to strong, on "trigger" points along the meridians. This pressure stimulates, calms, and/or harmonizes the functions of both body and mind. It thus promotes and results in relaxation and reduction of stress. Shiatsu, by manipulation of pressure points along the meridians, balances the body's energy flow and eliminates energy blockages.

Swedish Massage

This type of massage is based on a technique developed in 1812 by Per Henrik Ling. In it, each part of the body is manipulated, through individual muscles, using percussive, tapping movements designed to stimulate the nervous system; a rolling movement of the fingers; and vibration of the body. A special formula of naturally enriched massage oil, which is beneficial to the skin, is used to reduce friction for smooth and gliding strokes. We suggest a heat pack, sauna, whirlpool bath, or a hot shower to warm up before this massage.

Reflexology

Early Chinese healers subscribed to the theory that the feet are, so to speak, the body's computer: all energy pathways throughout the body converge in the feet, and a specific reflex point in the feet corresponds to each organ of the body. Reflexology uses pressure, rubbing, pulling, and massage of the proper points of the feet and ankles to release blockages in the corresponding organ. Kinesiology, the science concerned with the interrelationship between physiological processes and anatomy with respect to movement, is also used, where indicated, to complement proper energy flow to achieve a feeling of well-being and aliveness.

Reflexology focuses on the reflex points of the feet. It was developed by William Fitzgerald in the 1900s in this country, but has been known in China as a healing therapy for many thousands of years. By applying firm pressure with the thumb to specific nerve endings in the foot, an impulse is conveyed which causes a reflex response. This stimulates body organs such as the pituitary glands, lungs, bladder, kidneys, stomach, and spleen to return to optimal functioning.

Athletic Massage

Athletic massage has been traced back to the Roman Empire. Athletes who participated in sports, and gladiators who engaged in physical combat, had a soothing massage after a long day of strenuous activity. To this day, top professional athletes keep their bodies finely tuned through massage. The theory of massage is that by working the whole body with deep penetrating strokes and by concentrating strokes on particular muscle groups, the muscles are stimulated and loosened. In addition, there is a therapeutic effect on problem areas.

Athletic massage is a very deep, penetrating massage, especially for the active person. Whatever the activity in which the client participates (jogging, tennis, swimming, cycling, golf, riding, skiing), this type of massage can be beneficial.

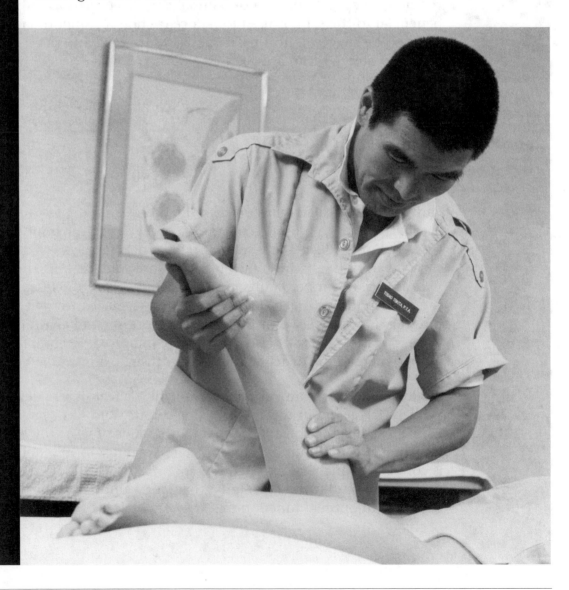

Underwater Pressure Massage

The therapeutic benefit of the underwater massage comes from the relaxing effect of warm water applied at variable force, particularly on deep-lying muscle layers, subcutaneous tissues, skin, and the abdominal organs (intestines).

In the underwater massage, the client lies relaxed in a large tub of warm water. A stream of water under pressure (ranging from 0.5 to a maximum of 7.0 bar absolute pressure units), is applied by means of a hose that has interchangeable nozzles.

Generally, the length of an underwater pressure massage is twenty to thirty minutes. It's necessary for the person to get used to the water for a

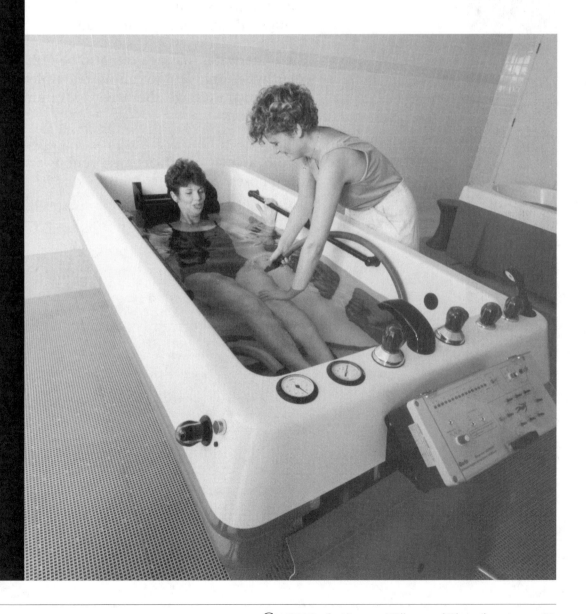

few minutes before starting the massage. After the massage, the client may want a cold affusion to stimulate circulation. The client should then rest for approximately thirty minutes.

Sensitive areas of the body, such as the spinous processes of the spinal column bone spurs, genitalia, anus, back of the knees, and the female breasts should be avoided during the underwater massage. Similarly, the massage is not recommended for any recent athletic injuries; open wounds; hematomas in an acute state; effusions in the knee joints; acute muscle, ligament, and tendon pulls; and recent fractures.

Indications: Fractures, osteosynthesis, dislocation, sprains, contusions in the subacute stages after a client has been released, sciatica, lumbalgia, brachialgia, joint and scar contractures, myogeloses, degenerative spinal disorders, chronic joint rheumatism, muscular rheumatism, Bechterev's Disease (ankylosing spondylitis), scoliosis, flaccid and spastic paralyses

The underwater massage can also be utilized for muscular hypertonia and for uninjured athletes as a warm-down massage after strenuous training and competition.

Contraindications: Cardiovascular insufficiencies, venous disorders, thromboses, varices

Manual Lymphatic Drainage (Massage)

MASSAGE THERAPIES

Definition: In the 1930s Dr. Emil Vodder publicized a light stroking massage, which he called lymph drainage massage. Since that time, manual lymphatic drainage (MLD) massage has developed into a medically applied method used in many instances. This is a non (skin) friction technique, which boosts the lymph drainage circulation system.

Indications: Skin ailments, pre- and post-surgery swelling, any soft tissue swelling, fibrocystic scarring, and pre-edema stages that prevent normal lymphatic flow

Contraindications: Any acute bacteriological or viral infection (common cold, influenza), thrombosis, malignant tumors, cardiovascular insufficiency, kidney malfunctioning

Effects: All tissue is drained via blood and lymphatic vessels. A sedating neurological effect causes the client to feel deeply relaxed. Lymphatic flow is promoted, and the body's immune system functions more effectively. The treatment is absolutely pain free and will not create any vascular lymphatic spasm.

Sound and Light Therapy

Definition:

A direct innate relationship exists between the seven colors of the spectrum, the seven notes of the musical scale, and the seven glandular systems of the body. Each color and note has a unique vibratory pattern, which stimulates in a corresponding manner the energy centers of the mind and the body.

Light from the sun enters the body through the eyes. The hypothalamus, a neuroendocrine gland, converts the electromagnetic signal of light into neurochemical impulses, which are then carried directly to the pituitary gland. The pituitary gland, in turn, secretes hormones, which stimulate the secretion of other hormones within the body, thereby maintaining homeostasis.

When the subconscious mind is exposed to pure vibration, either pure color or pure sound, the neuroendocrine and immune systems are purified. Pure color and sound also stimulate the ecstasy center of the brain by triggering the secretion of endorphins, powerful natural opiates. In this way, music and color create the experience of healing. Music and color have immense power on integrating and expanding the mind, and thus affect healing of the mind-body complex. True healing constitutes a positive, permanent transformation of mind with a resultant change in attitude, feeling, and behavior.

Effects:

Music and color, via the hypothalamus, have a direct effect on the thymus gland. This explains the beneficial effects music and color have in reducing unaccommodated stress. Unaccommodated stress suppresses the thymus gland and reduces your life energy.

The thymus gland is responsible for:

1. Immunological surveillance and the production of special T cells (the availability of a sufficient number of T cells determines whether you are resistant to disease)

2. The strength of muscular contractions

3. The flow of lymph (which is the body's cellular cleaning fluid) throughout the body, and regulating the life force that is flowing in and through your body moment by moment

The thymus gland is the center of your life energy. A healthy, active thymus gland creates vibrant and positive health. Thus, music and color can stimulate and enhance the proper functioning of the thymus gland.

MASSAGE THERAPIES

Ayurveda

Ayurveda, which means "the science of healthy living" in Sanskrit, is a holistic system of health principles which was developed and perfected in India thousands of years ago. Because it is a science, Ayurveda does not belong to India or the East, but is Vedic, or true for all times and places. It is a timely addition to the American treatment repertoire since it offers, with diligence and humility, the possibility of a healthy life for all.

Although Ayurveda is recognized as the earliest form of scientific medical knowledge, the exact historical beginning is at present unknown. The presumed time period ranges from 10,000 to 2,000 B.C. One of the most comprehensive attempts to describe the science of Ayurveda in Western terms was Dr. J. F. Royle's lectures delivered at King's College, London, in 1837. His series was entitled "On the Antiquity of Hindu Medicine."

Dr. Royle, a former Bengal army medical officer, shows the Ayurvedic roots in the knowledge of medicinal plants, biochemistry, and therapeutics used by Arabian, Greek, and Tibetan physicians. He outlines his historical connection among Charaka, the great Ayurvedic physician, Avicenna, the Arabic healer, and Hippocrates of Greece. In fact, Hippocrates introduced Ayurveda to the West in his humoral medicine, which, in essence, is the Ayurvedic theory of constitutional pathology—the parent of all medical systems.

According to Ayurveda, the human constitution—as well as the entire environment—is composed of five basic elements: earth, water, fire, air, and space. In an ideal situation, these five basic elements exist in a perpetual dynamic harmony, creating life, good health, and the perfection that is living creation. Ayurveda undergoes a further theoretical refinement when it identifies the functional triad known as the Tridosha, or three great basic factors governing human life (water, fire, and air). The constant interplay of these three great fundamental forces is described in Ayurveda as the theory of the Tridoshas. Healing occurs when the dynamic harmony of the doshas is restored. Disease can only occur when there is an abnormal affliction, an imbalance, in one, two, or all three elements.

Ayurvedic knowledge has flowed freely through the Far East, the Middle East, and Renaissance Europe, and exhibits a working harmony with all forms of native and folk medicines. Thanks to the work of great and highly principled Ayurvedists such as Dr. Vasant Lad and Dr. Chandrasekar Thakkur, Americans are at last adopting Ayurveda. Finally being recognized as the original holistic health system, Ayurveda emphasizes wellness and prevention, as well as disease management and cure.

Cranial-Sacral Therapy

Pioneered by William G. Sutherland in the 1920s, cranial-sacral therapy is a branch of osteopathy specializing in the study of the bones of the skull (cranium) and their relationship to ill health. It involves gently guiding and releasing tensions through very mild pressure on the different cranial bones near the sutures of the skull, where one bone lies next to another. Cranial-sacral therapy is reported effective in treating headaches, chronic ear infection, deafness, sinusitis, facial pain, and lower back pain.

Feldenkrais Method

Russian-born Israeli educator Moshe Feldenkrais based this method on the importance of awareness in human functioning. Feldenkrais consists of two branches: awareness through movement and functional integration. Feldenkrais believed awareness had to be achieved through experiences, not taught verbally. To that end, participants accomplish movements and postures they think unattainable, producing greater vitality. Functional integration involves treating the nervous system primarily through the skeletal structure, by using hands-on, painless manipulation.

Hellerwork

Founded in 1979 by Joseph Heller in the United States, the major components comprising Hellerwork include: deep-tissue body work affecting the nervous and muscular systems; movement re-education training to learn how to experience the full manifestation of spirit; and video feedback to view how we accomplish simple acts of daily life.

Treatments are offered in an eleven-session series, with each treatment consisting of one-hour of body work and thirty minutes of movement.

Trager Work

This body work therapy was developed by American medical practitioner Dr. Milton Trager in the 1920s. It makes extensive use of touch-contact, and encourages the patient to experience the "freeing up" of different parts of the body. The technique consists of simple exercises called Mentastics and deep nonintrusive hands-on work. The idea is to use motion in the muscles and joints to produce positive sensory feelings, which are then fed back into the central nervous system. The result is a feeling of lightness, freedom, and flexibility.

Watsu

Watsu is a body work technique that incorporates the moves and stretches of shiatsu while the client is in water. It began when Harold Dull of the School of Shiatsu and Massage at Harbin Hot Springs started floating people and then applying the Zen shiatsu techniques he studied in Japan. Watsu has now spread around the world, and developed into a powerful form which massage therapists find alleviates a wide range of physical and emotional conditions.

Jin Shin Jyutsu

A gentle, hands-on ancient healing art, Jin Shin Jyutsu allows the flow of energy to be restored by releasing blockages through touch. Jin Shin Jyutsu's origins are in Japanese Kojiki documents of the seventh century. Master Joro Maurai popularized this technique in the early 1920s.

In a typical session, which lasts about one hour, the client remains fully clothed, lying on his or her back. The practitioner identifies energy blocks by listening to the pulse and then holding two points in combination to release blockages.

Ortho-Bionomy

This system of body work was developed by Arthur Lincoln Pauls, a British osteopath, in the 1970s. It is homeopathic in principle. Ortho-Bionomy loosely translates from the Greek as the "correct application of the laws of life."

Gentle, relaxing movements and comfortable postures are used to ease the body into positions that unlock tensions and release stressful muscular patterns. This technique is nonintrusive, nonforceful, and encourages natural structural realignment and balance.

Reiki

Reiki is a Japanese word that is literally translated as "universal life force energy." It is an energy therapy whose roots can be traced back six thousand years. Although of ancient origin, it is one of the most widely practiced forms of alternative healing today, and practitioners can be found in many countries around the world. There are several forms of Reiki training, with the Traditional Usui School (named for founder Dr. Mikao Usui) being the most popular.

Reiki is extremely effective in helping individuals to release blockages and imbalances in their energetic bodies (mental, physical, emotional, and spiritual). Reiki may affect change in the chemical structure of the body as well as help create mental balance. The outcomes are different for every treatment.

Reiki has been effective in treating many stress-related illnesses, including anxiety, asthma, arthritis, back pain, cancer, carpal tunnel syndrome, headaches, irritable bowel syndrome, knee pain, muscular aches, post-surgical trauma, temporomandibular joint (TMJ) syndrome, toothaches, and many others too numerous to list. It is also complementary to other forms of healing, including traditional (allopathic) medicine, acupuncture, chiropractic, cranial-sacral therapy, massage therapy, and so on. Some doctors and many nurses in hospitals around the United States, as well as elsewhere in the world, have been trained in Reiki.

Anyone who desires to become a Reiki practitioner can do so by participating in an attunement process with a Reiki master. Once attunded an individual is always connected to the Reiki energy. The attunement is necessary in the same manner that a radio needs to be tuned to a particular station in order to receive a specific broadcast.

Rolfing

Rolfing is a technique developed to re-order the major body segments. Swiss-born biochemist Dr. Ida Rolf founded Rolfing in the 1940s. It was further developed in the 1960s in the United States. Rolfing utilizes a deep-tissue massage technique to bring head, shoulders, thorax, pelvis, and legs into vertical alignment. It allows more efficient use of the muscles with less expended energy by lifting the head and chest and lengthening the body's trunk. A sense of lightness and greater mobility often result.

Treatments are offered in a ten-session series, as well as additional advanced sessions.

CHAPTER 7

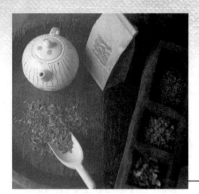

STEAM VAPOR BATH AND SAUNA

Steam Vapor Bath

Definition: Heating water to a high temperature produces the gaseous state of water. Wet or dry (sauna) steam is invaluable in stimulating the skin and the resultant perspiration helps to evacuate stored toxins.

Equipment: Boiling kettle, electric home vaporizer, or cold steam humidifier

Indications: Sinus attacks, breathing problems, bronchitis, hoarseness, laryngitis

Procedure: Prepare vaporizer.

Add a few drops of compound or simple tincture of benzoin to the vaporizer lid. (The tincture is made from a resin, so it will leave a gummy film, but it is very helpful in chest complaints, and has the added advantage of being a cosmetic aid. It is also a remarkable aid in restoring the voice.)

In the event there is no electric vaporizer available, boil water in a kettle, and keep it going by means of an electric tray, or some other safe arrangement.

Create an improvised tent over the client's body and direct the steam so that the client does not get too wet or perspire. A large umbrella can be used.

Occasionally sponge, or use a cold mitten massage on, the client's body, as this will aid circulation and create a feeling of well-being.

> **WARNING**
>
> Since water must be hot before it turns to steam, it must be handled very cautiously. Test and check each step in any of these suggested procedures to ensure personal safety.

Facials

To duplicate a professional facial, follow this procedure. This procedure is most useful for those with excessively oily skin. Do it in a non-drafty area to avoid chilling.

Procedure:

Bring to a vigorous boil in a Pyrex pot two quarts of water to which two tablespoons of chamomile tea have been added.

Remove the pot from the heat, place a newspaper on a table, and place the hot pot on the paper.

Sit with your face above the pot (but not close enough to get burned).

Improvise a tent by surrounding your head and the pot with a towel so that no steam escapes. Sit under the tent with eyes closed for five to ten minutes, breathing with your mouth open.

The pores of the face will open and perspiration will pour out.

Afterward, gently push out the blackheads with a cotton swab.

Close the pores with a splash of cold water, and sweep face with a cotton pad moistened with an herbal astringent, such as witch hazel.

Hot Steam Bath

Definition: A free flow of perspiration will often relieve the extreme pain of arthritis, gout, and sciatica, and will ease other pain. Steam baths are often available in local gyms, and are now available in steam rooms or pre-built sauna units for home.

Indications: Arthritis, fractures, sprains, sciatica, chronic low back pains, eliminates stored toxins

Finnish Sauna

Definition: Many accident victims or arthritis clients find that the dry heat of the Finnish sauna helps them to function in a more normal manner. There is an intense but tolerable heat in the sauna room, and this causes profuse perspiration within a few minutes. The ideal way to take a sauna is to perspire, then take a tepid or a cool shower, and then plunge into a cold pool of water. The total effect of these three water activities is a feeling of great cleanliness and exhilaration.

Indications: Fatigue, arthritis, after exercise, rheumatism, skin problems, poor circulation

The body soon develops a capacity to tolerate frequent saunas.

WARNING

Control the tendency for headache or dizziness by applying a cold compress to the forehead.

CHAPTER 8

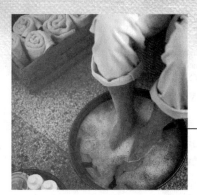

WATER AFFUSIONS

Affusions

Kneipp considers affusions a characteristic hydrotherapeutic treatment. One typical feature of affusions is the precise regulation of the direction of the water stream on the body. Affusions have a tonic effect. There are both simple affusions, making use of a stream of water without pressure, and affusions under pressure. Thus, there are two factors to consider in calculating the amount of stimulus: thermal and mechanical.

Kneipp claims that the water should surround the body like a coat. The primary effect of an affusion under pressure is mechanical. In simple affusions the temperatures used are extremely cold. In certain circumstances there can be an alternation of lukewarm and hot affusions. As in the case of all hydrotherapeutic uses of water, the patient's body and especially the feet should be warmed before and after the cold affusions. The length of the affusion depends on the individual reaction of each part of the body. A uniform reddening of the skin should take place.

Knee Affusion—
Cold Temperature

WATER AFFUSIONS

Indications: Vascular headaches, poor blood circulation in legs, elevated body temperature, varicose veins

Contraindications: Menstruation, sciatic pain, bladder or kidney infection, cold feet, oversensitivity to cold, low blood pressure

Equipment: 3/4 inch hose, 3 1/2 feet long

Effects: Reduces blood pressure, increases arterial blood flow, stimulates venous blood flow, helps relieve insomnia

Procedure:

1. **Cold Knee Affusion, Back Side**
   Temperature: 65°F

   The client inhales and exhales evenly during the beginning of the cold affusion.

   The affusion begins on the outside part of the right foot.

   Hose upwards along the calf three to four inches above the popliteal space (the back part of the leg behind the knee).

   Maintain position until the skin turns red, then move downwards inside the calf to the heel.

   Direct the hose at the left popliteal space and switch from left popliteal space to right, then back to left.

   Then hose down the inside of the left calf to the heel.

   Move to the front side.

2. Cold Knee Affusion, Front Side
Temperature: 65°F

The client breathes evenly while the cold affusion begins on the outside of the foot.

Hose the front part of the leg upwards three to four inches to the kneecap.

Stay in place until the skin turns red, then hose downwards inside the calf to the toes.

Repeat the same stroke on the left leg. Continue the affusion above the knee and switch from left kneecap to the right one and back again.

Then hose downwards inside the left calf to the toes.

Conclude with circular affusion on the bottom of both feet.

Wipe water off with hands. Do not towel dry.

The affusion should be followed by active exercise.

The legs should be kept warm by having the client exercise or wear socks in bed.

Knee Affusion—
Alternate Temperature

Indications: Vascular headaches, poor blood circulation in the legs, elevated body temperature, chronic cold feet

Contraindications: Menstruation, sciatic pain, bladder or kidney infection, varicose veins, low blood pressure, persistent chills

Effects: Reduces blood pressure, increases arterial blood flow, relaxes, relieves insomnia

Equipment: 3/4 inch hose, 3 1/2 feet long

Procedure:

1. **Warm Affusion, Back Side**
   Temperature: 97–100°F

   Start on the outside part of the right foot.

   Hose upwards along the calf (one hand width above the popliteal space).

   Maintain position until the client feels warm and a light redness of the skin appears.

   Continue downwards inside the calf.

   Repeat the same stroke on the left leg.

   Move to the front side.

   Warm Affusion, Front Side
   Temperature: 97–100°F

   Start on the outside part of the right foot.

   Hose the front part of the leg upwards (one hand width above the kneecap).

   Maintain position until the client feels warm and a light redness of the skin appears.

   Continue downwards inside the calf.

   Repeat the same stroke on the left leg.

Proceed with cold affusion.

2. **Cold Affusion, Back Side**
Temperature: 65°F

The client inhales and exhales evenly while the cold affusion begins on the outside of the right foot.

Hose upwards along the calf to one hand width above the kneecap.

Hose across the popliteal space then downwards inside the calf.

Repeat the same stroke on the left leg.

Move to the front side

Cold Affusion, Front Side
Temperature: 65°F

The client inhales and exhales evenly while the cold affusion begins on the outside of the right foot.

Hose the front part of the leg upwards (to one hand width above the kneecap).

Hose across the kneecap, then downwards inside the calf.

Repeat the same stroke on the left leg.

3. Repeat Warm Affusion.

4. Repeat Cold Affusion.

5. Finish with cold circular affusion on the bottom of both feet.

Wipe off water with both hands. Do not towel dry.

Have client rest for one hour and keep the body warm.

Leg Affusion—Cold Temperature

Indications: Unstable cardiovascular system, varicose veins, poor blood circulation in legs

Contraindications: Menstruation, oversensitivity to cold, sciatic pain, bladder or kidney infection, cold feet, low blood pressure

Effects: Reduces blood pressure, increases arterial blood flow, stimulates venous blood flow, relaxes

Equipment: $3/4$ inch hose, $3^1/2$ feet long

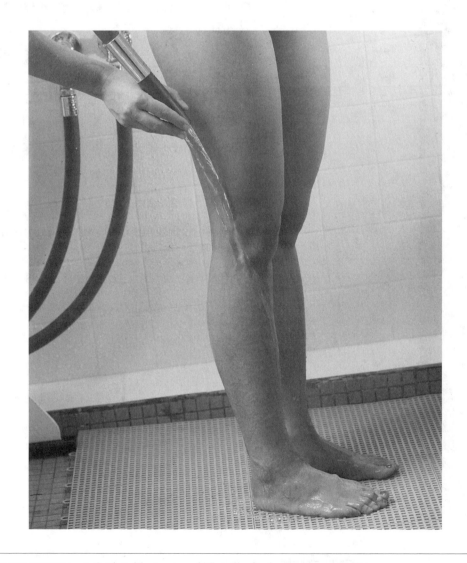

WATER AFFUSIONS

Procedure:

1. **Cold Leg Affusion, Back Side**
   Temperature: 65°F

   The client inhales and exhales evenly while the cold affusion begins on the outside of the right foot.

   Hose upwards along the outside of the leg to the gluteus. Maintain position until skin reddens, then move downwards inside the leg to the heel.

   Repeat the same stroke on the left leg but stay with the affusion on the gluteus and switch from left side to right and back to the left side.

   Then continue hosing downwards inside the left leg to the heel.

   Move to the front side.

2. **Cold Leg Affusion, Front Side**
   Temperature: 65°F

   The client inhales and exhales evenly while the cold affusion begins on the outside of the right foot.

   Hose upwards on the front part of the leg to the inguinal space. Maintain position until the skin appears red, then move downwards inside the leg to the toes.

   Repeat the same stroke on the left leg, but continue affusion on the inguinal space and switch from left side to right then to left side again.

   Continue hosing downwards inside the left leg to the toes.

   Conclude with cold circular affusion on the bottom of both feet.

   Wipe off water with hands. Do not towel dry.

   The affusion should be followed by active exercise or one hour of bed rest.

Leg Affusion— Alternate Temperature

Indications: Poor blood circulation, insomnia

Contraindications: Menstruation, sciatic pain, bladder or kidney infection, oversensitivity to cold

Effects: Reduces blood pressure, enhances blood circulation, increases arterial blood flow, stimulates venous blood flow, relaxes

Equipment: $3/4$ inch hose, $3^1/2$ feet long

Procedure:

1. **Warm Affusion, Back Side**
   Temperature: 97–100°F

   Start on the outside of the right foot.

   Hose upwards along the outside of the leg to the gluteus.

   Maintain the hose position until the client feels warm and the skin reddens.

   Continue down the inside of the leg to the toes.

   Repeat the same stroke for the left leg.

   Move to the front side.

   Warm Affusion, Front Side
   Temperature: 97–100°F

   Start on the right outside of the right foot.

   Hose up along the outside of the leg to the inguinal space.

   Maintain the hose position until the client feels warm and a light redness of the skin appears.

Continue down the inside of the leg to the toes.

Repeat the same stroke on the left side.

Proceed with cold affusion.

2. Cold Affusion, Back Side
Temperature: 65°F

The client inhales and exhales evenly while the cold affusion begins on the outside of the right foot.

Hose up along the lateral part of the leg to the gluteus.

Maintain hose position (but not for as long as the warm affusion).

Continue down the inside of the leg.

Repeat the stroke on the left side.

Move to the front side.

Cold Affusion, Front Side
Temperature: 65°F

The client inhales and exhales evenly while the cold affusion begins on the outside of the right foot.

Hose up along the outside of the leg to the inguinal space.

Maintain hose position.

Continue downwards inside the leg to the toes.

Repeat the same stroke on the left side.

3. Repeat Warm Affusion, Front Side.

4. Repeat Cold Affusion, Back Side.

5. Finish with cold circular affusion on the bottom of both feet.

Wipe off the water with hands.

Have client rest for one hour. Make sure the body stays warm.

Full Body Affusion—
Cold Temperature

Indications: Weak immune system

Contraindications: Menstruation, sciatica, bladder or kidney infection, chronic cold feet, oversensitivity to cold, arteriosclerosis, blood pressure disorders

Effects: Stabilizes vegetative nervous system, increases metabolic rate, increases blood circulation

Equipment: Shower hose

Procedure:

1. Cold Affusion, Back Side
Temperature: 65°F

Client inhales and exhales evenly while the cold affusion begins on the right foot.

Hose up along the leg to the gluteus, then down inside the leg to the heel. Hose up from the left foot along the leg to the gluteus. Move from the gluteus to the right hand.

Move up the right arm to the shoulder.

Move down the spine on the right side.

Move from under the gluteus to the left hand.

Move up the left arm to the shoulder, then switch from left side to right and back to left side again.

Move down spine on the left side to the gluteus, then down the inside of the left leg to the heel.

> ### *NOTE:*
> Before you start this treatment, have client splash water on forehead and chest. Treatment should be done after a dry sauna, whirlpool, steam sauna, or aroma bath.

2. Cold Affusion, Front Side
Temperature: 65°F

Client inhales and exhales evenly while the cold affusion begins on the right foot.

Hose up the front part of the leg to the inguinal space.

Move down the inside of the leg to the toes.

Hose up the front part of the left leg to the inguinal space.

Move from the inguinal space to the right hand, then to the shoulder.

Move down the right side of the sternum to the inguinal space.

Move to the left hand, then up the left arm to the shoulder.

Hose the left side, then the right, and back to the left side. Move down the left side of the sternum.

Hose the abdomen clockwise, then down the inside of the left leg to the toes.

Finish with a cold circular affusion on the bottom of both feet.

Wipe off the water with hands. Do not towel dry.

The affusion should be followed with rest.

Arm Affusion—
Cold Temperature

Indications: Fatigue, heart palpitations, low blood pressure

Contraindications: Coronary heart ailments, asthma

Effects: Refreshing, stimulates blood flow

Equipment: Shower hose

> **NOTE:**
>
> Do not start this treatment if client has cold hands.

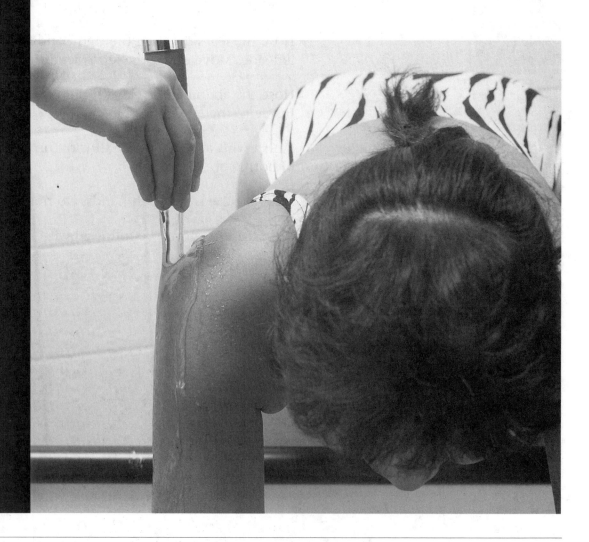

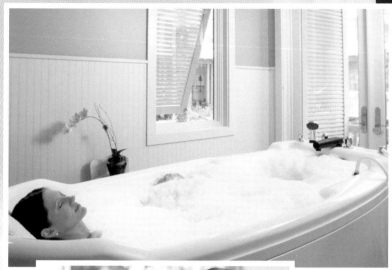

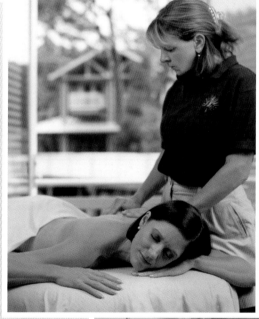

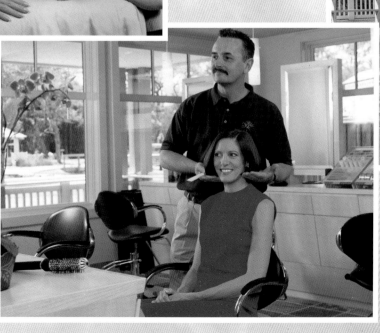

Spa Member Directory 2002

SPA MEMBER DIRECTORY 2002

■ Type of Spa	□ Salon Services	▨ Retail			
□ Spa Treatments	▨ Medical Affiliation	□ Other			
▨ Beauty Services	□ Programs				

- Day Spas listed in *COLOR* and *LARGER TYPE* have applied for and received accreditation by The Day Spa Association.
- Spa members marked with ✈'Year' are proud recipients of the "Distinguished Day Spa of the Year Award."

SPA NAME	ADDRESS	PHONE/FAX	EMAIL/WEBSITE	DAY SPA	SALON w/SPA SERVICES	WELLNESS CENTER	AFFILIATED w/HEALTH CLUB	AFFILIATED w/MEDICAL FACILITY	SPA RESORT/DESTINATION	LIFESTYLE STORE	
CALIFORNIA – NORTH											
A Simple Touch Spa	239 Center St. Healdsburg, CA 95448	707-433-6856 f: 707-433-6873	smtchspa@iosl.net **asimpletouchspa.com**	•							
Aesthetic Profiles	990 Sonoma Ave., Ste. 2A Santa Rosa, CA 95404	707-523-0893 f: 707-579-0459	facial@sonic.net **aesthetiProfiles.com**	•							
AXIS Personal Trainers and SPA	536 N. Santa Cruz Ave. Los Gatos, CA 95030	408-399-7521 f: 408-399-7531	ssaxe@axispt.com **axispt.com**				•				
AXIS Personal Trainers and SPA	544 N. San Antonio Rd. Mountain View, CA 94040	650-229-1100 f: 650-229-0990	aselman@axispt.com **axispt.com**				•				
Atzen Skin Care Center	281 E. Hamilton Ave., Ste. 9 Campbell, CA 95008	408-370-SKIN f: 408-370-4755	**atzen.com**	•							
Blue Sky Day Spa	4250 H St., Ste. 1 Sacramento, CA 95819	916-455-6200 f: 916-455-6255	cajay@sacweb.com **blueskydayspa.com**	•							
Body Spa	222 W. Lockeford St., Ste. 5 Lodi, CA 95240	209-367-5800 f: 916-689-8444	bodyspa2001@yahoo.com **bodyspadayspa.com**	•		•					
Caress Day Spa	911 Capitola Ave. Capitola, CA 95010	831-462-4422 f: 831-462-0296	marilee@scruznet.com **caressdayspa.com**	•							
HARMONIE-EUROPEAN DAY SPA	14501 Big Basin Way Saratoga, CA 95070	408-741-4997 f: 408-741-4901	pbottero@harmoniespa.com **harmoniespa.com**	•							
La Concha Spa Salon	1042 Lincoln Ave. San Jose, CA 95125	408-286-8612 f: 408-288-6472	Relax@laconchaspa.com **laconcha.com**	•							
Massage Masters Day Spa	14025 Ventura Blvd. Sherman Oaks, CA 91423	818-990-1076 f: 818-990-1161	sgroce@massagemasters.com **massagemasters.com**					•			
PRESTON WYNNE SPA AND SALON SUCCESS SYSTEMS ✈1999	14567 Big Basin Way Saratoga, CA 95070	408-741-5525 f: 408-741-4903	dayspa@prestonwynne.com **prestonwynne.com**	•							
re:fresh, a day spa	1130 Post St. San Francisco, CA 94109	415-563-2316 f: 415-445-9310		•							
Sabrina's Day Spa	170 Farmer's Ln. Santa Rosa, CA 95405	707-568-5620 f: 707-568-5624	info@sabrinasdayspa.com **sabrinasdayspa.com**	•							
St. James Studio	8300 Fair Oaks Blvd., No. 306 Carmichael, CA 95608	916-944-7361 f: 916-944-7361	SJSPA@hotmail.com	•							
Violet Johnson's Wellness Spa	1314 Lincoln Ave., Ste. 2F San Jose, CA 95014	408-297-4899 f: 408-297-4899	vjwellness@aol.com **vjwellness.com**	•	•						
Wolf Mountain Day Spa	15690-B Johnson Pl. Grass Valley, CA 95949	530-477-2340 f: 530-477-2364	simplyah@jps.net	•							
CALIFORNIA – SOUTH											
A Day Spa.com	325 W. Washington St. San Diego, CA 92103	619-293-3093	adayspa@hotmail.com **adayspa.com**	•							
A New Beginning	138 N. Lake Ave. Pasadena, CA 91101	626-449-1231 f: 626-449-1235	**newbeginningspa.com**	•				•			
All About Massage	74-121 Hwy. 111 Palm Desert, CA 92260	760-346-7949 f: 760-346-4549	aboutmassg@aol.com **allaboutmassage.com**	•	•	•					•
Allen Edwards Serenity Spa	20855 Ventura Blvd., Ste. 6 Woodland Hills, CA 91364	818-593-7094 f: 818-884-3615	lisa@allenedwards.com	•	•						
Amadeus Spa	799 East Green St. Pasadena, CA 91101	626-578-3404 f: 626-356-9757	amadeusnpb@slashcom.net **amadeusspa.com**	•	•						
Amadeus Spa	978 Avocado Ave. Newport Beach, CA 92660	949-718-9588 f: 949-718-0462	amaspanb@pacell.net **amadeusspa.com**	•	•						
Aveda Spa at Kriza	19524 Nordhoff St., No. 8-11 Northridge, CA 91324	818-772-2040 f: 818-772-6696	**kriza.com**	•							
Beauty Kliniek Aromatherapy Day Spa & Wellness Center	3268 Governor Dr. San Diego, CA 92122	858-457-0191 f: 858-457-0378	info@beautykliniek.com **beautykliniek.com**	•	•						
BELLISSIMA DAY SPA	122 E. Grand Ave. Escondido, CA 92025	760-480-9072 f: 760-480-9851	spa@connect.com **bellissima-spa.com**	•	•						
Bonnie's Hair Stop (under development)	33315 Hwy. 215 South Menifee Valley, CA 92584	909-672-1964									
DuBunné Massage Centre	23725 Arlington Ave. Torrence, CA 90501	310-326-9062 f: 310-326-7056	Info@dubunne.com **dubunne.com**	•							
Enessa - Aromatherapy Wellness Spa	8012-1/2 Melrose Ave. Los Angeles, CA 90046	888-4-ENESSA f: 323-932-7059	enessa@pacbell.net **enessa.com**	•							
Euphoria (opening 2002)	6262 Cathedral Oaks Rd. Santa Barbara, CA 93117	805-683-0359	lclausen@attglobal.net	•		•					
Expressions Day Spa	5101 Ocean Front Walk Marina del Rey, CA 90292	310-306-2285 f: 310-577-9664	ExpressionDaySpa@aol.com **hometown.aol.com/expressiondayspa**	•							
Gaia Day Spa	1299 Prospect St., Ste.105 La Jolla, CA 92037	858-456-8797 f: 858-455-9396	gaiadayspa@gaiadayspa.com **gaiadayspa.com**	•							

Columns (left to right):
1. MASSAGES
2. CRANIAL MASSAGE
3. REIKI / SHIATSU
4. LA STONE / HOT STONE
5. LYMPH DRAINAGE
6. PREGNANCY TREATMENTS
7. REFLEXOLOGY
8. POLARITY
9. FACIALS
10. NON-SURGICAL FACE LIFT
11. MICRODERMABRASION
12. CHEMICAL PEELS
13. BODY PACKS / HERBAL WRAPS
14. BODY TONING / CONTOURING
15. EXFOLIATION
16. CELLULITE
17. ENDERMOLOGY
18. ARYURVEDA
19. HEAT TREATMENTS
20. AROMATHERAPY
21. HYDROTHERAPY / VICHY SHOWER
22. ACUPUNCTURE
23. OXYGEN THERAPY
24. ELECTROLYSIS
25. LASER HAIR REMOVAL
26. WAXING / SUGARING
27. MAKEUP CONSULTATION
28. PERMANENT MAKEUP
29. SPA MANICURE / PEDICURE
30. SCALP TREATMENTS
31. SPA HAIR CARE
32. PLASTIC SURGEON
33. DERMATOLOGIST
34. CHIROPRACTIC
35. HOMEOPATHIC OTHER
36. WEIGHT MANAGEMENT
37. NUTRITIONIST
38. FITNESS CLASSES
39. FITNESS EQUIPMENT
40. PERSONAL TRAINERS
41. YOGA / MEDITATION
42. LECTURES / WORKSHOPS
43. BODY / BATH / HAIR / SKIN
44. AROMATHERAPY
45. COSMETICS
46. SPA CLOTHING
47. GIFT CERTIFICATES
48. GIFT ITEMS
49. NUTRITIONAL SUPPLEMENTS
50. A-LA-CARTE SERVICES
51. PACKAGES
52. BRIDAL PACKAGES
53. MEN SPECIFIC TREATMENTS
54. FENG SHUI TESTED SPACE
55. STEAM / SAUNA
56. LOCKER ROOM
57. LOCKER ROOMS FOR MEN
58. PVT. TREATMENT ROOMS
59. MEETING / PARTY ROOM
60. PARKING
61. ACCOMMODATIONS NEARBY

#	1	2	3	4	5	6	7	8	9	10	11	12	13	14	15	16	17	18	19	20	21	22	23	24	25	26	27	28	29	30	31	32	33	34	35	36	37	38	39	40	41	42	43	44	45	46	47	48	49	50	51	52	53	54	55	56	57	58	59	60	61
R1								•		•				•	•					•		•	•			•	•		•	•	•						•						•	•	•		•	•													
R2	•				•	•		•	•	•	•	•			•		•			•						•	•		•	•			•										•	•	•		•	•		•	•	•		•						•	
R3	•					•		•						•						•						•														•	•			•				•	•		•			•				•	•	•	
R4	•					•		•						•						•						•														•	•		•	•				•	•		•			•				•	•	•	
R5	•				•			•						•						•						•														•	•		•					•						•	•					•	•	
R6	•	•						•						•						•	•					•	•		•	•													•	•	•	•	•			•	•			•				•		•	•
R7	•	•						•						•						•	•																•	•						•	•	•		•										•		•	•
R8	•		•	•			•							•	•	•			•	•	•					•	•	•															•	•	•	•	•		•	•	•	•			•				•		•	•
R9	•		•	•	•	•	•	•					•	•	•	•	•	•	•	•	•	•	•	•	•	•	•		•	•													•	•	•	•	•	•	•	•	•	•	•		•	•	•		•		•	•
R10	•			•			•							•					•	•	•	•				•	•		•	•	•													•	•	•	•	•	•	•	•	•			•	•		•	•	•	•	•
R11	•			•	•	•	•						•	•	•	•	•	•	•	•	•				•	•	•		•	•	•		•						•	•	•	•	•	•	•	•	•	•	•	•	•	•	•		•			•	•		•	•
R12	•					•	•	•						•						•	•											•				•							•	•	•	•	•		•	•	•	•	•						•	•	•	•
R13	•	•												•				•		•																	•						•		•	•	•	•	•	•				•				•		•	•
R14	•		•	•			•							•	•	•	•	•	•	•	•	•																				•	•		•	•	•	•	•	•	•	•	•					•		•	•
R15	•		•	•	•	•								•	•	•	•	•	•	•	•					•	•	•	•	•	•	•					•						•	•	•	•	•	•	•	•	•	•	•				•		•	•
R16	•		•	•	•	•								•				•	•	•	•	•	•			•					•		•	•					•	•	•	•	•	•	•	•	•	•	•	•	•	•	•		•				•		•	•
R17	•		•	•	•	•								•				•		•	•											•		•								•	•	•	•	•	•	•	•	•	•						•		•	•	•

SPA MEMBER DIRECTORY 2002

	Type of Spa		Salon Services		Retail
	Spa Treatments		Medical Affiliation		Other
	Beauty Services		Programs		

- Day Spas listed in *COLOR* and *LARGER TYPE* have applied for and received accreditation by The Day Spa Association.
- Spa members marked with 'Year' are proud recipients of the "Distringuished Day Spa of the Year Award."

SPA NAME	ADDRESS	PHONE/FAX	EMAIL/WEBSITE	DAY SPA	SALON w/SPA SERVICES	WELLNESS CENTER	AFFILIATED w/HEALTH CLUB	AFFILIATED w/MEDICAL FACILITY	SPA RESORT/DESTINATION	LIFESTYLE STORE	SPA RESTAURANT
CALIFORNIA – SOUTH (continued)											
Gauthier Total Image Spa	14449 Ventura Blvd. Sherman Oaks, CA 91423	818-501-4423 f: 818-995-7256	info@gauthierspa.com **gauthierspa.com**	•							
GLEN IVY HOT SPRINGS SPA	25000 Glen Ivy Rd. Corona, CA 91719	800-454-8772 f: 909-277-1202	mkatgihs@aol.com **glenivy.com**	•							
Harmony Skin Care & Day Spa	31 W. Sierra Madre Blvd. Sierra Madre, CA 91024	626-836-1061 f: 626-836-1063	harmonyspa@earthlink.net **citydirect.com/harmonyskincare**	•							
International Skin & Body Care	325 Cajon St. Redlands, CA 92373	909-793-9080 f: 909-307-2788	intldayspa@aol.com **intldayspa.com**	•							
Le Meridian Spa	22224 La Palma Ave., Ste. C Yorba Linda, CA 92887	714-692-1902 f: 714-692-1922	info@lemeridian.net **lemeridian.net**	•							
Le Petite Retreat	331 N. Larchmont Blvd. Los Angeles, CA 90004	323-466-1028 f: 323-462-4008	lepetiteretreat@aol.com	•		•					
L'Onie Health & Wellness Day Spa	7643 Girard Ave. La Jolla, CA 92037	858-456-8663 f: 858-456-8089	lonie4@aol.com **lonie.com**	•		•					
Manaois'	401 Bluff Rd. Montebello, CA 90640	310-287-8552	TessM99@aol.com								
Medi Touch Clinical Skin Care & Day Spa	5216 W. Bordeaux Ct. Visalia, CA 93291	559-734-2400 f: 559-688-6744	zulh786@aol.com	•							
Metropolis Body Spa	115 W. Main St., Ste. B Visalia, CA 93291	559-622-0208 f: 559-733-7365			•						
Sk Sanctuary La Jolla	6919 La Jolla Blvd. La Jolla, CA 92037	858-459-2400 f: 858-459-2442	kellysk@hotmail.com							•	
Skin Solutions	4510 Executive Dr., No. 405 San Diego, CA 92121	858-622-0656	c_naor@hotmail.com **skinsolutionscenter.com**							•	
Skinsational Skin Day Spa	300 Carlsbad Village Dr., Ste. 201B Carlsbad, CA 92008	760-434-8118 f: 760-434-1597	**skinsationalspa.com**	•					•		
The Greenhouse - Beverly Hills	417 N. Canon Dr. Beverly Hills, CA 90210	310-274-6417 f: 310-274-3207	**thegreenhousespa.com**	•							•
The Greenhouse - Newport Beach	401 Newport Center Dr., Ste. 216 Newport Beach, CA 92660	949-644-4677 f: 949-644-6614	**thegreenhousespa.com**	•	•						
The Massage Therapy Center	2130 S. Sawtelle Blvd., Ste. 207 Los Angeles, CA 90025	310-444-8989 f: 310-479-5039	**massagenow.com**								
The Oaks at Ojai	122 East Ojai Ave. Ojai, CA 93023	805-646-5573 f: 805-646-8382	Sheila@oaksspa.com **oakspa.com**							•	
The Palms at Palm Springs	572 N. Indian Canyon Dr. Palm Springs, CA 92262	805-646-5573 f: 805-646-8382	Sheila@oaksspa.com **oakspa.com**							•	
The Skin Spa	17401 Ventura Blvd. Encino, CA 91316	818-995-3888 f: 818-995-3048	Theskinspa@aol.com **skinspa.com**	•	•	•					
The Spa at the Sporting Club at Aventine	8930 University Center Ln. San Diego, CA 92122	858-713-1866 f: 858-552-8264	dana.wilkerson@clubone.com **thesportingclub.com**	•			•				
Vera's Retreat in the Glen	2980 Beverly Glen Circle, Ste.100 Bel Air, CA 90077	310-470-6362 f: 818-779-0955	angelabrown@verasdirect.com **verasretreat.com**	•							
NEW YORK – CITY											
ATZEN MEDI-SPA 2001	856 Lexington Ave. New York, NY 10021	212-517-2400 f: 212-861-6971	**atzen.com**	•							
Body Essentials Day Spa & Ayurvedic Center	11 W. 36th St. New York, NY 10018	212-465-2220 f: 212-947-7720	bodyess@aol.com **bodyessentials.com**	•	•						
CARAPAN URBAN SPA & STORE	5 W. 16th St., Garden Level New York, NY 10011	212-633-6220 f: 212-929-3342	carapan@aol.com **carapan.com**	•						•	
Dr. Margolin's Wellness Spa	166 Fifth Ave., 2nd Fl. New York, NY 10010	212-675-9355 f: 212-675-9381	margoctr@aol.com **drmargolins.com**	•	•						
FELINE DAY SPA	235 W. 75th St. New York, NY 10023	800-FELINE-1 f: 212-579-8145	**felinedayspa.citysearch.com**	•	•						
Juva Medi-Spa	60 E. 56th St. New York, NY 10022	212-688-5882 f: 212-421-9502	mail@juvaskin.com **juvaskin.com**						•		
Oasis Day Spa	108 E. 16th St. New York, NY 10003	212-254-7722 f: 212-505-3560	nydayspa@aol.com **nydayspa.com**	•							
Skin Deep Luxury Day Spa and Well-Being Center for Men & Women	2071 Clove Rd. Staten Island, NY 10304	718-720-6383 f: 718-818-0421	SkinDeepSpa@aol.com **skindeepspa.com**	•	•						
SPA F.L.A.M.	309 E. 75th St., Ste. 8 New York, NY 10021	212-988-3181	karenflam@yahoo.com **spaflam.com**	•							
The Greenhouse - New York	127 E. 57th St. New York, NY 10022	212-644-4449 f: 212-644-3044	**greenhousespa.com**	•							
THE STRESS LESS STEP	115 E. 57th St., 5th Fl. New York, NY 10022	212-826-6222 f: 212-826-1010	**stresslessstep.com**	•		•					

Column headers (read top-to-bottom, left-to-right):

1. MASSAGES
2. CRANIAL MASSAGE
3. REIKI / SHIATSU
4. LA STONE / HOT STONE
5. LYMPH DRAINAGE
6. PREGNANCY TREATMENTS
7. REFLEXOLOGY
8. POLARITY
9. FACIALS
10. NON-SURGICAL FACE LIFT
11. MICRODERMABRASION
12. CHEMICAL PEELS
13. BODY PACKS / HERBAL WRAPS
14. BODY TONING / CONTOURING
15. EXFOLIATION
16. CELLULITE
17. ENDERMOLOGY
18. ARYURVEDA
19. HEAT TREATMENTS
20. AROMATHERAPY
21. HYDROTHERAPY / VICHY SHOWER
22. ACUPUNCTURE
23. OXYGEN THERAPY
24. ELECTROLYSIS
25. LASER HAIR REMOVAL
26. WAXING / SUGARING
27. MAKEUP CONSULTATION
28. PERMANENT MAKEUP
29. SPA MANICURE / PEDICURE
30. SCALP TREATMENTS
31. SPA HAIR CARE
32. PLASTIC SURGEON
33. DERMATOLOGIST
34. CHIROPRACTIC
35. HOMEOPATHIC OTHER
36. WEIGHT MANAGEMENT
37. NUTRITIONIST
38. FITNESS CLASSES
39. FITNESS EQUIPMENT
40. PERSONAL TRAINERS
41. YOGA / MEDITATION
42. LECTURES / WORKSHOPS
43. BODY / BATH / HAIR / SKIN
44. AROMATHERAPY
45. COSMETICS
46. SPA CLOTHING
47. GIFT CERTIFICATES
48. GIFT ITEMS
49. NUTRITIONAL SUPPLEMENTS
50. A-LA-CARTE SERVICES
51. PACKAGES
52. BRIDAL PACKAGES
53. MEN SPECIFIC TREATMENTS
54. FENG SHUI TESTED SPACE
55. STEAM / SAUNA
56. LOCKER ROOM
57. LOCKER ROOMS FOR MEN
58. PVT. TREATMENT ROOMS
59. MEETING / PARTY ROOM
60. PARKING
61. ACCOMMODATIONS NEARBY

	Type of Spa		Salon Services		Retail
	Spa Treatments		Medical Affiliation		Other
	Beauty Services		Programs		

- Day Spas listed in *COLOR* and *LARGER TYPE* have applied for and received accreditation by The Day Spa Association.
- Spa members marked with "Year" are proud recipients of the "Distringuished Day Spa of the Year Award."

SPA NAME	ADDRESS	PHONE/FAX	EMAIL/WEBSITE	DAY SPA	SALON w/SPA SERVICES	WELLNESS CENTER	AFFILIATED w/HEALTH CLUB	AFFILIATED w/MEDICAL FACILITY	SPA RESORT/DESTINATION	LIFESTYLE STORE	SPA RESTAURANT
NEW YORK STATE											
A-Nu-U Spa	45 Quaker Ave., Ste. 201 Cornwall, NY 12518	845-534-3656 f: 845-569-1671	info@anuuspa.com **anuuspa.com**	•							
Bodicures Ltd.	735 E. Boston Post Rd. Mamaroneck, NY 10543	914-777-2873 f: 914-381-2579	bdcures@aol.com	•							
DeFranco Spagnolo Salon/Day Spa	200 Middle Neck Rd. Great Neck, NY 11021	516-466-6752 f: 516-466-2618	softcurly@DFSSalon.com **dfssalon.com**	•							
ENHANCE FACE & BODY SPA	100 N. Central Park Ave. Hartsdale, NY 10530	914-997-8878 f: 914-997-8148	susan@enhancespa.com **enhancespa.com**	•							
Eva of Sweden Body & Beauty Center	Marriott Hotel, Rt. 119 Tarrytown, NY 10591	914-631-6111	spawish2.com/evaofsweden.htm	•			•				
Garrison Golf Club Sports+Spa	P.O. Box 348/2015 Rt. 9 Garrison, NY 10524	845-424-3604 f: 845-424-3586	jendirito@garrisongolfclub.com **garrisongolfclub.com**	•	•		•	•			•
Gurney's Inn Resort & Spa	290 Old Montauk Hwy. Montauk, NY 11954	631-668-2509 f: 631-668-3689	gurneysinn@aol.com **gurneys-inn.com**						•		
Healthy by Nature	126 Laurel Rd. East Northport, NY 11731	631-757-3366 f: 631-757-3385	drcjnd@hotmail.com **healthybynature.com**			•					
Luna Mesa Day Spa	225 Montauk Hwy., Ste. 14-15 Moriches, NY 11955	631-874-4114 f: 631-874-4844	massagework@aol.com **lunamesa.com**	•							
Haven	6464 Montgomery St. Rhinebeck, NY 12572	845-876-7369 f: 845-876-7629	luxspa@aol.com				•				
Nothing But The Best Day Spa	45 Rt. 347 Mount Sinai, NY 11776	631-473-8055 f: 631-473-8972	nbtbspa@aol.com	•							
Phases Skin Spa	180 E. Main St., Ste. 226 Smithtown, NY 11787	516-361-7650 f: 516-361-7638	phases@phasesskincare.com **phasesskincare.com**	•							
Phases Skin Spa	97F Main St. Stony Brook, NY 11790	631-751-1511 f: 631-751-2333	phases@phasesskincare.com **phasesskincare.com**	•							
Professional Touch Day Spa	11 West St. Warwick, NY 10990	845-987-8951 f: 845-986-7952	ferenz@warwick.net	•							
Riverspa	50 S. Buckhout St. Irvington, NY 10533	914-591-5757 f: 914-591-4256		•		•					
The Greenhouse - Manhasset	1950 Northern Blvd., A2 Manhasset, NY 11030	516-869-0100 f: 516-869-0177	**thegreenhousespa.com**	•							•
NORTHEAST											
ADAM BRODERICK SALON & SPA 2001	89 Danbury Rd. Ridgefield, CT 06877	203-431-3994 f: 203-431-4156	eileen@adambroderick.com **adambroderick.com**	•	•	•		•		•	•
DERMA CLINIC EUROPEAN DAY SPA	299 Post Rd. East, Playhouse Sq. Westport, CT 06881	203-227-0771 f: 203-454-5877		•							
Solei Day Spa + Tanning	222 Greenwood Ave. Bethel, CT 06801	203-744-7385 f: 203-778-2162	soleispa@aol.com **soleispa.com**	•							
The Greenhouse - Greenwich	44-48 Putnam Ave. Greenwich, CT 06830	203-622-0300 f: 203-622-0644	**thegreenhousespa.com**	•							
The Spa at Huntington	101 Country Pl. Shelton, CT 06484	203-926-6050	debblisk@snet.net	•							
Élan Vitál - Rejuvenating Spa and Ayurvedic Medical Center	7 Whittier Pl., Ste.108 Charles River Park/ Boston, MA 02114	617-227-6573 f: 508-770-0618	ayurveda@hotmail.com **ayurvedausa.net**	•				•			
Elizabeth Renee Esthetics	26 Grove St. Wellesley, MA 02482	781-237-SKIN f: 781-237-2593	erespa@aol.com **erespa.com**	•							
Sage Club Spa	140 Great Plain Ave. Wellesley, MA 02181	781-239-6066 f: 781-239-6087		•							
SpringRain DaySpa Face & Body Spa	475 Winter St. Waltham, MA 02451	781-895-0010 f: 617-332-9866	SpringRainspa@aol.com	•							
Windkist Medical Laser Aesthetics and Day Spa	168 N. Main St. Andover, MA 01810	978-623-3200 f: 978-685-3195	EliasGlob@aol.com		•						
Stars Esthetics Spa	6245 Falls Rd., 2nd Level Baltimore, MD 21209	410-832-0002 f: 410-832-5282	pattea5@starspa.com **starsspa.com**	•							
Cameo Visage Inc. Day Spa Essentials	5301 Buckeystown Pike, Ste.102 Frederick, MD 21704	301-620-2617 f: 301-831-6759	CamVinFo@aol.com	•							
The Grand View Inn & Resort	580 Mountain Rd. Jaffrey, NH 03452	603-532-9880 f: 603-532-6252	thegrandviewinn@aol.com **grandviewinn.com**						•		
Avanti Salon & Spa	345 Rt. 9 South Manalapan, NJ 07726	732-780-0222 f: 732-780-0266	vlAvanti@aol.com **avantisalonspa.com**	•	•	•					
BEAUTY SPA AT ENGLEWOOD	363 Grand Ave. Englewood, NJ 07627	201-567-6020 f: 201-568-7567		•				•			

The column headers (left to right) are:

1. MASSAGES
2. CRANIAL MASSAGE
3. REIKI / SHIATSU
4. LA STONE / HOT STONE
5. LYMPH DRAINAGE
6. PREGNANCY TREATMENTS
7. REFLEXOLOGY
8. POLARITY
9. FACIALS
10. NON-SURGICAL FACE LIFT
11. MICRODERMABRASION
12. CHEMICAL PEELS
13. BODY PACKS / HERBAL WRAPS
14. BODY TONING / CONTOURING
15. EXFOLIATION
16. CELLULITE
17. ENDERMOLOGY
18. ARYURVEDA
19. HEAT TREATMENTS
20. AROMATHERAPY
21. HYDROTHERAPY / VICHY SHOWER
22. ACUPUNCTURE
23. OXYGEN THERAPY
24. ELECTROLYSIS
25. LASER HAIR REMOVAL
26. WAXING / SUGARING
27. MAKEUP CONSULTATION
28. PERMANENT MAKEUP
29. SPA MANICURE / PEDICURE
30. SCALP TREATMENTS
31. SPA HAIR CARE
32. PLASTIC SURGEON
33. DERMATOLOGIST
34. CHIROPRACTIC
35. HOMEOPATHIC OTHER
36. WEIGHT MANAGEMENT
37. NUTRITIONIST
38. FITNESS CLASSES
39. FITNESS EQUIPMENT
40. PERSONAL TRAINERS
41. YOGA / MEDITATION
42. LECTURES / WORKSHOPS
43. BODY / BATH / HAIR / SKIN
44. AROMATHERAPY
45. COSMETICS
46. SPA CLOTHING
47. GIFT CERTIFICATES
48. GIFT ITEMS
49. NUTRITIONAL SUPPLEMENTS
50. A-LA-CARTE SERVICES
51. PACKAGES
52. BRIDAL PACKAGES
53. MEN SPECIFIC TREATMENTS
54. FENG SHUI TESTED SPACE
55. STEAM / SAUNA
56. LOCKER ROOM
57. LOCKER ROOMS FOR MEN
58. PVT. TREATMENT ROOMS
59. MEETING / PARTY ROOM
60. PARKING
61. ACCOMMODATIONS NEARBY

Columns 1–23

#	1	2	3	4	5	6	7	8	9	10	11	12	13	14	15	16	17	18	19	20	21	22	23
1	•	•	•	•		•		•		•				•					•	•			
2	•			•		•	•		•										•	•			
3	•			•		•	•		•				•	•	•	•	•		•	•			
4	•		•	•		•	•		•					•				•		•			
5	•			•		•	•	•		•	•	•	•		•					•			
6	•		•	•		•			•	•	•									•			
7	•		•	•	•	•	•		•	•	•		•	•	•				•	•	•	•	
8	•									•		•	•							•		•	
9	•	•			•				•				•	•	•				•				
10	•	•		•	•	•	•	•	•	•		•	•	•	•				•	•	•		
11	•	•	•			•			•										•	•			
12										•		•	•							•	•	•	
13	•				•				•				•	•	•		•		•				
14	•		•	•	•	•	•	•	•		•		•		•				•		•		
15	•						•			•			•								•		
16	•		•	•	•	•	•	•	•	•	•	•	•	•	•	•	•	•	•	•	•		

Columns 24–42

#	24	25	26	27	28	29	30	31	32	33	34	35	36	37	38	39	40	41	42
1			•			•												•	•
2	•	•	•	•		•	•	•											
3	•	•	•	•		•	•	•											
4			•	•	•	•	•	•											
5						•	•					•							
6	•	•	•	•		•	•	•						•	•	•	•		
7												•	•	•					
8	•	•	•			•	•					•							
9			•	•		•	•			•							•	•	
10			•	•		•	•		•										
11	•	•	•																
12	•	•	•	•													•		
13	•	•	•			•	•												
14			•		•	•	•										•		
15						•	•	•	•	•	•	•		•	•	•	•	•	•
16	•	•	•	•		•	•	•		•									

Columns 43–61

#	43	44	45	46	47	48	49	50	51	52	53	54	55	56	57	58	59	60	61
1	•				•	•		•	•	•			•				•		•
2	•	•	•		•	•							•					•	•
3	•	•	•					•	•		•					•		•	
4	•	•	•	•	•	•					•		•				•		•
5	•	•				•				•			•			•		•	•
6	•	•	•	•	•	•	•	•	•	•	•	•	•	•	•	•	•	•	•
7						•							•					•	•
8	•	•	•		•	•											•	•	
9	•	•	•	•	•	•		•	•				•						•
10	•	•	•		•	•		•	•	•								•	•
11	•	•	•		•	•		•	•									•	•
12	•	•	•		•	•		•					•			•		•	•
13	•	•	•	•	•	•		•			•							•	•
14	•	•	•		•	•		•	•		•	•	•					•	•
15					•	•	•											•	•
16	•	•	•		•	•		•	•	•			•			•		•	•

SPA MEMBER DIRECTORY 2002

Type of Spa | Salon Services | Retail
Spa Treatments | Medical Affiliation | Other
Beauty Services | Programs

- Day Spas listed in *COLOR* and *LARGER TYPE* have applied for and received accreditation by The Day Spa Association.
- Spa members marked with 'Year' are proud recipients of the "Distringuished Day Spa of the Year Award."

SPA NAME	ADDRESS	PHONE/FAX	EMAIL/WEBSITE	DAY SPA	SALON w/SPA SERVICES	WELLNESS CENTER	AFFILIATED w/HEALTH CLUB	AFFILIATED w/MEDICAL FACILITY	SPA RESORT/DESTINATION	LIFESTYLE STORE	SPA RESTAURANT
NORTHEAST (continued)											
DEPASQUALE, THE SPA ⟶2000	Rt. 10 East, Powder Mill Plaza, Morris Plains, NJ 07950	973-538-3811 f: 973-359-8940	thespa@bellatlantic.net **depasqualethespa.com**			●		●			
International Salon & Spa	25 Sparta Ave., Sparta, NJ 07871	973-729-9037 f: 973-729-2746	joedi@nac.net	●							
Phases Skin Spa	2033 Lemoine Ave., Fort Lee, NJ 07024	201-585-9797 f: 201-585-1501	phases@phasesskincare.com **phasesskincare.com**	●							
Serenity Day Spa	330 Old Bridge Tpk., South River, NJ 08882	732-257-8118 f: 732-257-5559	**serenitydayspanj.com**	●							
Spa Serein	Woodcliff Lake Hilton, 200 Tice Blvd., Woodcliff Lake, NJ 07675	201-505-0273 f: 201-634-8692		●	●				●		●
THE BRASS ROSE SPA & SALON	26 Rt. 94, Blairstown, NJ 07825	908-362-9009 f: 908-362-9040	rose@brassrose.com **brassrose.com**	●							
The Fountain European Spa	1100 Rt. 17 North, Ramsey, NJ 07446	201-327-5155 f: 201-327-4243	fountain@nis.net **fountaineuropeanspa.com**	●							
The Spa at 800 West	800 W. Rt. 70, Marlton, NJ 08053	856-985-9800 f: 856-985-3347	Spa@800west.com **800west.com**	●					●		
Vito Mazza Salon & Day Spa	114 Main St., Woodbridge, NJ 07095	732-636-0119 f: 732-636-3391	vito@vitomazza.com **vitomazza.com**	●							
Day Spa at Botta Aesthetic Surgery	KF Bldg., 5168 Campbells Run Rd., Pittsburgh, PA 15205	412-788-8011 f: 412-788-8411	BASurgery@aol.com **pittsburgh.net/Botta**	●	●			●			
Lady Di's Salon & Spa	100 E. Glenolden Ave., B-26, Glenolden, PA 19036	610-461-6400 f: 610-461-1743	info@ladydispa.com **ladydispa.com**	●							
Spa at Felicita	550 Lakewood Dr., Harrisburg, PA 17112	717-599-5301 f: 717-599-7353	**Felicitaresort.com**	●					●		
Spa Maison	305 Horsham Rd., Horsham, PA 19044	215-675-2887 f: 215-675-6881	info@spamaison.com **spamaison.com**	●	●						
Spa Uptown	1 Chatham Center, Pittsburgh, PA 15219	412-281-5400		●							
Technicolor Salon + Day Spa	3017 W. Tilghman St., Allentown, PA 18017	610-821-8921 f: 610-821-8546		●							
Topper's Spa	117 S. 19th St., Philadelphia, PA 19103	215-496-9966	corporate@toppersspa.com **toppersspa.com**	●							
Kenneth Coté Renewal Center	333 Main St., East Greenwich, RI 02818	401-884-2810 f: 401-785-9808	kencotespa@aol.com **kennethcote.com**	●							
New Life Hiking Spa (Inn of the Six Mountains)	P.O. Box 395, Killington, VT 05751	802-422-4302 f: 802-422-4321	hikingspa@aol.com **newlifehikingspa.com**						●		
Europa Salon	709 Beechurst Ave., Morgantown, WV 26505	304-292-2554 f: 304-292-3424	EdeBeaute@aol.com		●						
Curves For Women	722 Foxcroft Ave., Martinsburg, WV 25401	304-263-4200 f: 304-263-4200	losso@intrepid.net curvesforwomen.com		●						
SOUTHEAST											
THE GREENHOUSE - BIRMINGHAM	240 Summit Blvd., Ste. 200, Birmingham, AL 35243	205-967-1177 f: 205-967-5793	**thegreenhousespa.com**	●							
The Spa at The Beach Club	453 Beach Club Trl., Gulf Shores, AL 36542	334-540-ASPA f: 334-540-2583	spa@beachclubal.com **beachclubal.com**							●	
Accardi, The Salon	4046 Park St., St Petersburg, FL 33710	727-343-1234			●						
Alpha Beauty Clinic Inc.	4131 Southside Blvd., Ste. 205, Jacksonville, FL 32216	904-998-9977 f: 904-998-9942	AlphaBeaut@aol.com	●							
Atzen Laboratories	1569 Main St., Dunedin/Tampa, FL 34698	888-GLYCO-10 f: 727-738-9193	**atzen.com**	●		●					
Bellazza Spa Salon & Boutique	72455 S.W. 57th Ct., Miami, FL 33143	305-284-0669 f: 305-665-3656	**bellaezzaspa.com**	●							
Body and Sole Day Spa	400 2nd St. North, Safety Harbor, FL 34695	727-725-3255 f: 727-725-2925	**bodyandsoledayspa.com**	●							
D. Laudati Salon at the Brazilian Court	301 Australian Ave., Palm Beach, FL 33480	561-833-7611 f: 561-471-9262	laudati@skybiz.com **dlaudatisalon.com**		●				●		
Danielle Spa for Beauty & Wellness	27160 Bay Landing Dr., Bonita Springs, FL 34135	941-947-5900 f: 941-495-9170		●							
Diva's Day Spa	4242 N. Federal Hwy., Ft. Lauderdale, FL 33308	954-771-9SPA(9772) f: 954-564-8145	divadayspa@aol.com **divadayspa.com**	●							
Holistic Treatments of Beauty	8501 S.W. 84th Ct., Miami, FL 33143	305-595-4806 f: 305-595-2133	phizoid@dnamail.com	●							
Irene's European Day Spa	628 Cleveland St., Ste. 300, Clearwater, FL 33755	727-462-8131 f: 727-367-0713	lrenesdayspa@mail.com **irenesdayspa.com**	●	●						

This table lists spa services (columns) against individual spas (rows). The column headers, read left to right, are:

1. MASSAGES
2. CRANIAL MASSAGE
3. REIKI / SHIATSU
4. LA STONE / HOT STONE
5. LYMPH DRAINAGE
6. PREGNANCY TREATMENTS
7. REFLEXOLOGY
8. POLARITY
9. FACIALS
10. NON-SURGICAL FACE LIFT
11. MICRODERMABRASION
12. CHEMICAL PEELS
13. BODY PACKS / HERBAL WRAPS
14. BODY TONING / CONTOURING
15. EXFOLIATION
16. CELLULITE
17. ENDERMOLOGY
18. ARYURVEDA
19. HEAT TREATMENTS
20. AROMATHERAPY
21. HYDROTHERAPY / VICHY SHOWER
22. ACUPUNCTURE
23. OXYGEN THERAPY
24. ELECTROLYSIS
25. LASER HAIR REMOVAL
26. WAXING / SUGARING
27. MAKEUP CONSULTATION
28. PERMANENT MAKEUP
29. SPA MANICURE / PEDICURE
30. SCALP TREATMENTS
31. SPA HAIR CARE
32. PLASTIC SURGEON
33. DERMATOLOGIST
34. CHIROPRACTIC
35. HOMEOPATHIC OTHER
36. WEIGHT MANAGEMENT
37. NUTRITIONIST
38. FITNESS CLASSES
39. FITNESS EQUIPMENT
40. PERSONAL TRAINERS
41. YOGA / MEDITATION
42. LECTURES / WORKSHOPS
43. BODY / BATH / HAIR / SKIN
44. AROMATHERAPY
45. COSMETICS
46. SPA CLOTHING
47. GIFT CERTIFICATES
48. GIFT ITEMS
49. NUTRITIONAL SUPPLEMENTS
50. A-LA-CARTE SERVICES
51. PACKAGES
52. BRIDAL PACKAGES
53. MEN SPECIFIC TREATMENTS
54. FENG SHUI TESTED SPACE
55. STEAM / SAUNA
56. LOCKER ROOM
57. LOCKER ROOMS FOR MEN
58. PVT. TREATMENT ROOMS
59. MEETING / PARTY ROOM
60. PARKING
61. ACCOMMODATIONS NEARBY

Row	1	2	3	4	5	6	7	8	9	10	11	12	13	14	15	16	17	18	19	20	21	22	23	24	25	26	27	28	29	30	31	32	33	34	35	36	37	38	39	40	41	42	43	44	45	46	47	48	49	50	51	52	53	54	55	56	57	58	59	60	61
1	•			•	•	•	•				•		•	•	•	•	•		•	•	•		•	•	•	•			•	•	•	•		•								•	•	•		•	•	•	•	•	•				•	•	•	•		•	•
2	•			•				•	•																•	•	•	•	•	•	•												•	•	•		•	•	•	•			•	•	•		•		•	•
3	•						•		•		•	•	•	•	•	•	•		•		•				•	•																	•	•			•	•	•	•		•	•	•		•		•	•
4	•						•		•			•	•	•	•	•	•		•	•					•	•			•	•	•												•	•	•		•	•	•	•		•	•	•		•		•	•
5	•	•					•	•		•										•						•			•	•	•		•						•	•	•		•						•	•			•	•	•	•	•	•	•	•
6	•		•	•			•			•		•							•	•						•	•		•	•	•												•	•	•	•	•	•	•	•			•	•	•		•		•	•
7	•		•	•	•					•		•							•	•						•	•		•	•	•												•	•	•	•	•	•	•	•			•	•	•		•		•	•
8	•		•	•			•		•			•							•	•						•	•		•	•	•												•	•	•	•	•	•	•	•	•		•	•	•			•	•	•
9	•		•	•			•		•				•	•	•	•		•	•	•						•	•		•	•	•												•	•	•	•	•	•	•	•			•	•	•		•		•	•
10	•		•	•			•	•		•	•		•	•	•	•	•	•	•	•						•	•		•	•	•	•					•	•	•		•		•	•	•	•	•		•	•	•	•			•	•	•		•	•	•
11	•		•		•				•			•	•	•	•	•	•	•	•	•				•		•	•					•					•	•					•	•			•	•	•	•			•	•	•		•		•	•
12	•	•	•	•					•			•										•					•																•		•			•	•				•	•	•	•	•	•		•	
13	•		•	•				•			•										•					•	•		•	•								•	•	•	•	•	•				•	•											•	
14	•		•	•					•																	•	•		•	•	•												•	•			•	•	•	•			•	•	•		•	•	•	•
15	•								•		•	•	•	•	•	•	•		•							•	•		•	•	•												•	•	•			•	•	•	•			•	•	•		•	•	•	
16	•			•			•			•										•						•	•		•	•	•												•			•	•	•	•			•	•	•		•	•	•	•
17	•		•				•		•				•		•	•	•		•	•						•	•		•	•	•												•	•	•	•	•	•	•	•			•	•	•		•	•	•	•
18	•			•					•											•						•	•		•	•												•	•	•		•	•	•	•			•	•	•		•		•	•
19	•					•			•				•							•		•														•		•	•	•		•		•			•			•		•	•	•	•		•	•	•	
20	•							•			•					•					•					•	•		•	•	•												•	•	•	•	•	•	•				•	•	•				•	•
21	•						•	•		•					•		•							•		•	•									•	•	•	•		•	•	•	•			•			•	•			•	•	•	•	•	•	•	•

Row-continued (lower block, rows 22+):

Row	1	2	3	4	5	6	7	8	9	10	11	12	13	14	15	16	17	18	19	20	21	22	23	24	25	26	27	28	29	30	31	32	33	34	35	36	37	38	39	40	41	42	43	44	45	46	47	48	49	50	51	52	53	54	55	56	57	58	59	60	61
22	•			•	•		•		•					•	•	•	•									•	•		•	•	•												•	•	•	•	•	•		•	•		•		•	•	•	•			
23	•				•				•				•		•					•	•					•			•	•								•	•	•		•	•	•	•	•	•	•						•	•	•	•		•	•
24	•				•	•			•				•	•		•	•			•	•			•	•	•			•	•													•	•	•			•	•		•	•				•			•	•
25	•			•	•	•			•			•	•	•		•	•			•	•					•	•		•	•		•	•				•					•						•	•	•		•	•			•			•	•
26																										•	•		•														•		•		•														
27	•	•	•				•																			•	•	•	•	•	•												•	•	•	•	•	•	•	•			•	•	•		•	•	•	•
28		•	•								•		•	•	•	•	•			•						•			•	•	•							•					•	•			•	•	•	•			•	•	•		•	•	•	•
29	•			•	•	•	•		•	•	•	•	•	•	•	•				•						•	•		•	•	•							•	•	•			•	•	•	•	•	•	•	•		•	•	•	•	•		•	•	•
30	•		•	•	•	•	•		•			•	•	•	•	•			•	•					•	•	•	•	•	•	•					•	•	•	•	•	•		•	•	•	•	•	•	•	•	•	•			•	•	•	•		•	•
31	•	•	•	•	•	•	•		•				•	•	•	•			•	•	•			•	•	•	•	•	•	•	•		•		•	•	•	•	•	•	•	•	•	•	•	•	•	•	•	•	•	•	•	•	•	•	•	•	•	•	•

Legend:
- Type of Spa
- Spa Treatments
- Beauty Services
- Salon Services
- Medical Affiliation
- Programs
- Retail
- Other

- Day Spas listed in *COLOR* and *LARGER TYPE* have applied for and received accreditation by The Day Spa Association.
- Spa members marked with ★ 'Year' are proud recipients of the "Distinguished Day Spa of the Year Award."

SOUTHEAST (continued)

SPA NAME	ADDRESS	PHONE/FAX	EMAIL/WEBSITE	DAY SPA	SALON w/SPA SERVICES	WELLNESS CENTER	AFFILIATED w/HEALTH CLUB	AFFILIATED w/MEDICAL FACILITY	SPA RESORT/DESTINATION	LIFESTYLE STORE	SPA RESTAURANT
Island Massage Store and Day Spa	5343 Gulf Dr., Unit 500, Holmes Beach, FL 34217	941-779-0066 f: 941-778-6982	spaisland@aol.com **holmesbeachchamberofcommerce**	•		•	•	•		•	•
Kaffee's Garden Spa	4100 S. Dixie Hwy., Ste. D, West Palm Beach, FL 33405	561-833-4483 f: 561-833-4222	**kaffeesgardenspa.com**	•							
Movement Improvement	4720 S.E. 15th Ave., No. 215, Cape Coral, FL 33904	941-540-9933 f: 941-540-9933									
The Greenhouse - Orlando	5601 Universal Blvd., Orlando, FL 32819	407-503-1244 f: 407-503-1233	**thegreenhousespa.com**	•							
The Morel European Spa	2767 E. Oakland Park Blvd., Ft. Lauderdale, FL 33304	800-822-6675 954-561-8799 f: 954-564-1825	spa@moreleuropeanspa.com **moreleuropeanspa.com**	•							
The Spa At Amelia Island Plantation	P.O. Box 3000, Amelia Island, FL 32035	904-261-6161 f: 904-277-5984	huttol@aipfl.com **aipfl.com**			•			•	•	•
Touch of Class Day Spa	10331 W. Sample Rd., Coral Springs, FL 33065	954-346-0666 f: 954-227-6707	noraforever@hotmail.com	•	•	•					
Treatments Aesthetic Center & Spa	501 Village Green Pkwy., Ste.18, Bradenton, FL 34209	941-792-9108 f: 941-794-8732	Ranie1@aol.com **treatments.net**	•				•			
Brigette's, The Beauty Center	797 Redland Dr., Jonesboro, GA 30238	770-471-0174 f: 770-471-0174	brigettes@netzero.net **brigettespa.com**	•							
Renew Day Spa & Wellness Center	4347 Shallowford Rd., Marietta, GA 30062	770-998-8592	Renewsspa@bellsouth.net **renewdayspa.com**	•							
Spa Sydell	10593 Old Alabama Connector, Atlanta, GA 30004	770-552-1880		•							
Spa Sydell	3060 Peachtree Rd. N.W., Atlanta, GA 30305	404-237-2505 f: 404-237-1408		•							
Spa Sydell	1259 Cumberland Mall, Atlanta, GA 30339	770-801-0804 f: 770-801-8710		•							
Spa Sydell	1165 Perimeter Center West, Atlanta, GA 30346	770-551-8999 f: 770-551-8659		•							
Spa Sydell	2255 Pleasant Hill Rd., Duluth, GA 30096	770-622-5580 f: 770-622-4149		•							
Travis Salon & Spa	895 Flat Shoals Rd., Conyers, GA 30094	770-929-1742 f: 770-929-1455	travisa@ebellsouthnet.com	•							
Allie's Figure & Day Spa	200 Point St., Houma, LA 70360	985-873-7032 f: 985-872-9844	Alliesspa@eatel.net		•						
Belladonna Day Spa	2900 Magazine St., New Orleans, LA 70115	504-891-4393 f: 504-891-1004	**belladonnadayspa.com**	•							
BETH'S WELLNESS CENTER AT THE HORSESHOE CASINO HOTEL	722 Horseshoe Blvd., Bossier City, LA 71111	318-949-6595 f: 318-949-6595	bobbeth96@aol.com **bethswellness.com**	•		•					
Bodyjoys Day Spa & Salon	3423 St. Charles Ave., New Orleans, LA 70115	800-331-7812 504-895-4400 f: 504-895-4600	bodyjoys@bellsouth.net	•							
Rose Spa & Fitness Center (Harrahs Shreveport Hotel)	401 Market St., Ste. 1240, Shreveport, LA 71101	318-429-6855	cgreub@Shreveport.harrahs.com **Shreveport.harrahs.com**						•	•	•
The Sapphire Spa & Retreat	20109 Knox Rd., Cornelius, NC 28031	704-987-0006	**sapphirespa.com**	•							
Thee Salon and Day Spa	650 S.W. Broad St., Southern Pines, NC 28387	910-692-9144 f: 910-692-6050			•						
Pure Reflections Spa for Wellness	915 Tate Blvd. S.E., Ste. 170, Hickory, NC 28602	828-345-0800 f: 828-345-0350	dayspa@twave.net **purereflections.com**					•			
RENAISSANCE EUROPEAN DAY SPA	860 Elm St., Fayetteville, NC 28303	910-484-9922 f: 910-484-9339	**renaissanceeuropeandayspa.com**	•		•	•	•		•	•
The Spa at Margo Blue	7903 Providence Rd., Ste.125, Charlotte, NC 28277	704-341-0922 f: 704-544-1119	margo@margoblue.com **margoblue.com**	•							
Spa at Ivanhoe	451 N. Jeffries Blvd., Walterboro, SC 29488	843-549-2550 f: 843-538-3337	khiott@lowcountry.com	•							
Faces DaySpa	1000 WM. Hilton Pkwy., No. 0-2, Hilton Head Island, SC 29928	888-443-2237 f: 843-785-6110	info@hhfaces.com **hhfaces.com**								
Just B Spa & Apothecary	230 Franklin Rd., Factory at Franklin, Franklin, TN 37060	615-599-0559 f: 515/599-0856	**JustBSpa.com**	•					•	•	
Bella Spazio	7671 S. Northshore Dr., Knoxville, TN 37919	865-670-0998 f: 865-670-8925	edbaker@aol.com **bellaspazio.com**		•						
Yana's Salon & Spa	788 W. Main St., Ste. A, Hendersonville, TN 37075	615-822-9551 f: 615-822-9185	YanaSalonSpa@aol.com **yanassalonandspa.com**	•	•						
Changes Hairstyling & Day Spa	710 W. 21st St., Norfolk, VA 23517	757-625-5300 f: 757-623-6986	Changes@pin.net		•						

This spa services matrix uses 35 columns (labeled 1–35 left to right) with the service name in the right-hand label column.

1	2	3	4	5	6	7	8	9	10	11	12	13	14	15	16	17	18	19	20	21	22	23	24	25	26	27	28	29	30	31	32	33	34	35	SERVICE
•	•	•	•	•	•	•	•	•	•	•	•	•	•	•	•	•	•	•	•	•	•	•	•	•	•	•	•	•	•	•	•	•	•	•	MASSAGES
							•					•											•							•					CRANIAL MASSAGE
		•									•	•																					•	•	REIKI / SHIATSU
•	•	•	•	•		•		•				•	•																	•	•		•	•	LA STONE / HOT STONE
	•		•	•		•			•	•		•	•										•	•			•	•		•	•		•	•	LYMPH DRAINAGE
		•				•		•	•	•		•	•	•													•	•		•	•		•	•	PREGNANCY TREATMENTS
•	•		•	•		•	•	•		•		•	•	•	•	•	•	•	•	•	•	•		•	•	•	•	•	•	•	•	•	•	•	REFLEXOLOGY
		•	•																								•						•	•	POLARITY
•	•	•	•	•	•	•	•	•	•		•	•	•									•	•	•	•	•	•	•	•	•	•	•	•	•	FACIALS
	•		•	•		•						•	•											•	•	•		•		•	•		•	•	NON-SURGICAL FACE LIFT
•		•		•		•						•													•	•		•	•		•		•	•	MICRODERMABRASION
•						•						•																					•	•	CHEMICAL PEELS
•	•	•	•		•	•	•	•		•			•	•			•	•	•	•	•	•		•	•	•	•		•	•	•	•	•	•	BODY PACKS / HERBAL WRAPS
	•	•	•			•		•			•	•	•	•										•	•	•	•		•	•		•	•	BODY TONING / CONTOURING
•	•	•	•		•	•	•	•	•	•	•	•	•	•	•	•	•		•	•		•		•	•	•	•		•	•	•	•	•	•	EXFOLIATION
	•	•	•			•		•		•		•	•	•										•	•	•	•		•	•	•	•	•	•	CELLULITE
		•	•			•			•		•	•	•	•										•	•	•	•		•	•	•	•	•	•	ENDERMOLOGY
		•	•								•	•												•	•	•	•		•	•	•	•	•	•	ARYURVEDA
		•				•		•			•	•	•	•		•	•	•	•	•		•		•	•	•			•	•		•	•	HEAT TREATMENTS
•	•		•	•	•		•		•	•	•	•	•			•	•	•	•	•	•	•		•	•	•	•	•	•	•		•	•	AROMATHERAPY
•	•	•	•	•			•			•	•	•	•			•	•	•	•	•	•	•		•	•	•	•		•					HYDROTHERAPY / VICHY SHOWER
	•						•	•															•											ACUPUNCTURE
						•						•																						OXYGEN THERAPY
•		•	•									•	•										•	•										ELECTROLYSIS
	•	•				•						•																						LASER HAIR REMOVAL
•	•	•	•	•	•	•	•	•	•		•	•	•	•	•	•	•	•	•	•	•	•		•	•	•	•		•	•	•	•	•	WAXING / SUGARING
•	•	•	•	•	•	•	•	•	•	•		•	•	•	•	•	•	•	•	•	•	•		•	•	•			•	•	•	•	•	MAKEUP CONSULTATION
						•						•														•								•	PERMANENT MAKEUP
•	•	•	•	•	•	•	•	•	•	•	•	•	•	•	•	•	•	•	•	•	•	•		•	•	•	•		•	•	•			SPA MANICURE / PEDICURE
•	•	•	•		•	•		•	•	•		•	•	•	•	•	•	•	•	•	•			•	•	•	•		•	•				SCALP TREATMENTS
•	•	•	•		•	•	•		•			•		•	•	•		•	•	•	•			•	•	•	•		•					SPA HAIR CARE
		•										•	•												•										PLASTIC SURGEON
•												•													•						•				DERMATOLOGIST
						•																		•	•										CHIROPRACTIC
																																	•	HOMEOPATHIC OTHER
						•				•		•	•												•		•							•	WEIGHT MANAGEMENT
•			•			•				•		•	•												•		•								NUTRITIONIST
						•				•		•															•							•	FITNESS CLASSES
						•			•	•		•													•		•							•	FITNESS EQUIPMENT
						•				•		•															•								PERSONAL TRAINERS
		•				•								•																				YOGA / MEDITATION
		•				•						•													•		•							•	LECTURES / WORKSHOPS
•	•	•	•	•	•	•	•	•	•	•	•	•	•	•	•	•	•	•	•	•	•	•		•	•	•	•	•	•	•	•	•	•	•	BODY / BATH / HAIR / SKIN
	•	•	•	•	•	•	•	•		•		•	•	•	•	•	•	•	•	•	•	•		•	•	•	•	•	•	•	•	•	•	AROMATHERAPY
•	•	•	•	•	•	•	•	•	•		•	•	•	•	•	•	•	•	•	•				•	•	•	•	•	•	•	•	•	•	COSMETICS
		•	•			•	•					•															•	•	•					SPA CLOTHING
•	•	•	•	•	•	•	•	•	•	•	•	•	•	•	•	•	•	•	•	•				•	•	•	•	•	•	•		•	•	GIFT CERTIFICATES
•	•	•	•		•	•	•	•	•	•		•	•	•	•	•	•	•	•	•				•	•		•	•	•	•		•	•	GIFT ITEMS
	•	•	•			•	•					•	•	•										•	•	•	•		•				•	NUTRITIONAL SUPPLEMENTS
•	•	•	•	•		•	•	•	•	•		•	•	•	•	•	•	•	•	•	•				•	•	•	•	•	•	•	•		•	A-LA-CARTE SERVICES
•	•	•		•		•	•	•	•	•		•	•	•	•	•	•	•	•	•	•			•				•	•	•	•	•	•	•	PACKAGES
•		•			•	•	•		•			•	•															•	•		•			•	BRIDAL PACKAGES
•	•	•				•			•	•		•	•													•			•	•	•	•	•	•	MEN SPECIFIC TREATMENTS
		•						•																		•								FENG SHUI TESTED SPACE
•	•	•	•	•		•	•		•		•	•	•	•	•	•	•	•	•	•		•		•	•	•	•		•		•			STEAM / SAUNA
•	•	•	•		•	•			•		•	•	•	•	•	•	•	•	•	•				•	•	•	•		•					LOCKER ROOM
•	•	•	•		•	•		•	•	•		•	•	•	•	•	•	•	•	•		•		•	•	•		•	•					LOCKER ROOMS FOR MEN
•	•	•		•		•			•	•		•	•	•	•	•	•	•	•	•				•	•	•		•	•					PVT. TREATMENT ROOMS
	•	•	•					•	•	•			•											•	•	•		•	•		•			MEETING / PARTY ROOM
•		•	•	•			•	•				•																•	•		•			PARKING
	•	•	•	•			•			•	•					•	•	•	•			•	•			•	•		•					ACCOMMODATIONS NEARBY

SPA MEMBER DIRECTORY 2002

- Type of Spa
- Spa Treatments
- Beauty Services
- Salon Services
- Medical Affiliation
- Programs
- Retail
- Other

- Day Spas listed in *COLOR* and *LARGER TYPE* have applied for and received accreditation by The Day Spa Association.
- Spa members marked with ▸Year' are proud recipients of the "Distinguished Day Spa of the Year Award."

MIDWEST

SPA NAME	ADDRESS	PHONE/FAX	EMAIL/WEBSITE	DAY SPA	SALON w/SPA SERVICES	WELLNESS CENTER	AFFILIATED w/HEALTH CLUB	AFFILIATED w/MEDICAL FACILITY	SPA RESORT/DESTINATION	LIFESTYLE STORE	SPA RESTAURANT
Comfort & Joy Wellness Spa	9868 Main St., Fairfax Sq. Fairfax, VA 22031	703-267-2333	comfortjoy.com	•		•					
Cynia European Day Spa	1430 Spring Hill Rd. McLean, VA 22101	703-821-2522 f: 703-821-1304	cynia.com		•	•					
Face Works Day Spa	8502 Patterson Ave. Richmond, VA 23229	804-740-5665 f: 804-741-7203	faceworks@msn.com **faceworksdayspa.com**	•							
La Beauté Naturelle	3608 Forest Dr. Alexandria, VA 22302	703-998-0003 f: 703-379-2468	lbn4u@aol.com **labeautenaturelle.com**	•							
Bettye O. Day Spa	5200 S. Harper Ave. Chicago, IL 60615	800-262-6104 f: 773-752-2613	BettyeODaySpa@Earthlink.com **BettyeODaySpa.com**	•							
Day Escape, The Ultimate Spa	150 E. Ogden Ave., 2nd Fl. Westmont, IL 60559	630-455-0660 f: 630-455-0669	ULTISPA@AOL.COM	•							
Rodica European Skin & Body Care Center	Watertower Pl., 845 N. Michigan Ave. Ste. 944E / Chicago, IL 60611	312-527-1459 f: 312-943-7241	rodica13@MW.ldsoline.com **facialandbodybyrodica.com**	•							
House of Bianco Beauty Concepts & Day Spa	1000 E. 80th Pl., Twin Towers South Merrillville, IN 46410	219-769-1010 f: 219-791-1061		•	•						
Renú Salon & Day Spa	10020 E. U.S. Hwy. 36 Avon, IN 46123	317-209-7368 f: 317-209-7374	Renu10020@aol.com		•						
SERENITY, THE REJUVENATING DAY SPA	7211 W. 95th St. Overland Park, KS 66212	913-341-0025 f: 913-341-2192	JmHohn@hotmail.com serenitydayspa.net	•							
THE LIGHT TOUCH	211 Clover Ln. Louisville, KY 40207	502-893-9595 f: 502-893-3048	Lilliam@lighttouchspa.com **lighttouchspa.com**	•							
Regina Webb Salon & Day Spa	1945 Scottsville Rd., Ste. C-4 Bowling Green, KY 42104	270-781-4676 f: 270-782-8231	top20rist@aol.com	•				•	•		
Allen May Salon	1687 Cantor Center North Cantor, MI 48187	734-981-8223 f: 734-981-6805			•						
Douglas J. Day Spa Salon	4663 Ardmore Okemos, MI 48864	517-349-5271 f: 517-349-6922	Salon@douglasj.com **douglasj.com**	•	•					•	
Linda Micheals Day Spa	36 Hawk Dr. Great Falls, MI 59404	406-727-3287 f: 406-727-3232			•						
Polished Outlook, Inc. Day Spa Salon Boutique	101 Washington St. Milford, MI 48381	248-685-9898 f: 248-685 2837	polout@tir.com **polishedoutlook.com**	•	•					•	
Tamara Institute de Beaute	32520 Northwestern Hwy. Farmington Hills, MI 48334	248-855-0474 f: 248-855-0155	**Tamaraspa.com**	•							
The Greenhouse - Troy	2800 Big Beaver Rd., Space MI58 Troy, MI 48084	248-614-8952 f: 248-614-8972	**thegreenhousespa.com**	•							
GB & Co. Beauty.Hair.Skin.Spa	80 37th Ave. South St. Cloud, MN 56301	320-253-4832	berdtoy@aol.com		•						
Just For Me, The Spa	110 S. Greeley St. Stillwater, MN 55082	651-439-4662 f: 651-430-3740	**justformespa.com**	•	•	•	•			•	
Rodica Facial Salon	681 E. Lake St., Ste. 257 Wayzata, MN 55391	612-475-3111		•							
SIMONSON'S SALON & DAY SPA	3507 Round Lake Blvd. Anoka, MN 55303	763-427-0761 f: 763-427-0358	info@simonsons.com **simonsons.com**	•							
Simonson's Salon & Day Spa	19336 Hwy. 169 Elk River, MN 55330	763-441-5999	info@simonsons.com **simonsons.com**	•							
SIMONSON'S SALON & DAY SPA	13744 83rd Way Maple Grove, MN 55369	763-494-4863 f: 763-494-8392	info@simonsons.com **simonsons.com**	•							
The Day Spa	7575 France Ave. South Edina, MN 55435	952-830-0100 f: 952-806-0943	dayspamn@aol.com **adayatthespa.com**	•							
Tom Schmidt Urban Retreat	1609 W. Lake St. Minneapolis, MN 55408	612-827-5595 f: 612-827-8960	UrbanRetreat@msn.com **tomschmidturbanretreat.com**	•	•						
Salon De Christé	3901 Mid Rivers Mall Dr. St. Peters, MO 63376	636-939-4105 f: 636-939-4107	promiselc@earthlink.net **salondechriste.com**	•	•						
Spa St. Charles	2440 Executive Dr., Ste. 100 St. Charles, MO 63303	636-498-0707 f: 636-498-0708	info@spastcharles.com **spastcharles.com**		•						
The Face & The Body	7736 Forsyth Blvd. St. Louis, MO 63105	314-725-8975 f: 314-726-6268	**faceandbodyspa.com**	•							
The Face & The Body	1765 Clarkson Rd. Chesterfield, MO 63017	636-532-2500	**faceandbody.com**		•						
Escape for a Day Spa	631 16th St. Gulfport, MS 39507	228-897-1770 f: 228-897-1748	**escapespa.cs.com**	•							
Charles Scott Salon and Spa	19025 Olde Lake Rd. Rocky River, OH 44116	440-333-7994 f: 440-333-5330	**charlesscott.com**	•							

MASSAGES	CRANIAL MASSAGE	REIKI / SHIATSU	LA STONE / HOT STONE	LYMPH DRAINAGE	PREGNANCY TREATMENTS	REFLEXOLOGY	POLARITY	FACIALS	NON-SURGICAL FACE LIFT	MICRODERMABRASION	CHEMICAL PEELS	BODY PACKS / HERBAL WRAPS	BODY TONING / CONTOURING	EXFOLIATION	CELLULITE	ENDERMOLOGY	ARYURVEDA	HEAT TREATMENTS	AROMATHERAPY	HYDROTHERAPY / VICHY SHOWER	ACUPUNCTURE	OXYGEN THERAPY	ELECTROLYSIS	LASER HAIR REMOVAL	WAXING / SUGARING	MAKEUP CONSULTATION	PERMANENT MAKEUP	SPA MANICURE / PEDICURE	SCALP TREATMENTS	SPA HAIR CARE	PLASTIC SURGEON	DERMATOLOGIST	CHIROPRACTIC	HOMEOPATHIC OTHER	WEIGHT MANAGEMENT	NUTRITIONIST	FITNESS CLASSES	FITNESS EQUIPMENT	PERSONAL TRAINERS	YOGA / MEDITATION	LECTURES / WORKSHOPS	BODY / BATH / HAIR / SKIN	AROMATHERAPY	COSMETICS	SPA CLOTHING	GIFT CERTIFICATES	GIFT ITEMS	NUTRITIONAL SUPPLEMENTS	A-LA-CARTE SERVICES	PACKAGES	BRIDAL PACKAGES	MEN SPECIFIC TREATMENTS	FENG SHUI TESTED SPACE	STEAM / SAUNA	LOCKER ROOM	LOCKER ROOMS FOR MEN	PVT. TREATMENT ROOMS	MEETING / PARTY ROOM	PARKING	ACCOMMODATIONS NEARBY
•		•				•		•				•		•			•	•	•	•						•	•	•	•	•					•	•	•	•		•	•	•		•	•	•		•	•	•		•	•		•			•	•
•			•			•		•		•		•	•	•	•	•		•	•						•	•	•	•	•										•	•	•		•	•	•	•				•				•		•	•	•
•		•	•		•	•	•	•	•	•		•	•	•	•			•	•						•	•		•	•											•	•	•	•	•	•	•	•	•		•	•		•		•		•	•
•	•	•		•	•	•		•	•	•		•	•	•	•			•	•				•	•	•	•	•														•	•	•															•	•
•		•	•	•		•		•	•				•	•	•				•	•								•	•												•	•	•	•	•	•	•	•	•	•	•	•			•	•	•	•
•				•	•			•				•	•	•	•				•									•	•	•											•				•	•			•		•				•			•	•
•			•			•		•				•	•	•	•			•	•						•	•		•	•												•	•	•	•	•	•		•	•	•		•	•	•				•	•
•				•				•		•		•	•	•					•	•					•	•		•	•												•				•	•		•	•	•				•		•		•	•
•								•											•							•		•	•							•			•		•				•			•	•		•			•	•	•			•
•	•		•	•	•	•		•		•		•	•	•	•				•	•					•	•	•	•	•												•	•	•		•	•		•	•	•			•				•	•	
•	•	•	•	•		•		•		•		•	•	•	•			•	•						•	•		•	•	•	•	•			•	•	•	•	•		•	•	•	•	•	•		•	•		•					•			•	•
•				•	•			•	•	•				•	•				•	•						•		•	•	•		•			•						•	•	•		•	•			•	•	•	•	•	•	•			•	•	
•			•	•		•		•		•		•	•	•	•				•	•						•															•	•	•		•	•	•	•	•	•							•		
•		•	•		•	•		•	•			•	•	•				•	•	•			•		•	•	•	•													•	•	•	•	•	•	•	•	•	•								•	•
•			•			•		•				•	•	•						•					•	•		•	•		•		•	•							•				•	•		•								•		•	•	
•	•		•	•	•	•	•	•	•	•	•	•	•	•	•			•	•						•	•		•	•		•	•		•	•							•	•	•	•	•	•			•						•	•	•		•	•
•	•		•	•	•	•		•				•	•	•	•			•	•						•	•		•	•			•		•								•	•	•	•	•	•			•	•				•				•	•
•		•	•	•		•		•	•	•		•	•	•	•			•	•	•				•		•	•		•	•	•											•	•	•	•	•	•		•	•					•			•	•	
•	•	•			•	•	•	•	•	•	•	•	•	•				•	•								•	•							•	•	•	•	•		•					•	•		•	•								•		
•						•		•																	•			•							•	•	•	•	•		•				•				•								•		
•		•	•			•	•	•	•	•	•	•	•	•					•				•		•	•																•		•		•	•			•	•				•			•	•	•
•			•	•		•		•		•				•	•			•	•	•					•	•	•	•	•													•	•	•	•	•	•	•	•	•	•						•		•	•
•		•	•	•		•		•		•		•	•	•	•				•	•					•	•		•	•	•											•	•	•	•	•	•		•									•		•	•
•	•		•	•		•		•		•		•	•	•	•			•	•						•	•		•	•		•											•	•	•		•	•	•	•	•				•				•	•	
•			•	•		•	•	•	•	•		•	•	•	•			•	•						•	•		•	•	•										•	•	•	•	•	•	•	•	•	•	•	•		•	•	•		•	•	•	•
•	•	•		•	•	•		•	•	•		•	•	•	•	•	•	•	•	•			•		•	•		•	•	•	•									•	•	•	•	•	•	•	•	•	•	•	•	•		•	•	•	•	•	•	•	•

SPA MEMBER DIRECTORY 2002

Type of Spa · Salon Services · Retail
Spa Treatments · Medical Affiliation · Other
Beauty Services · Programs

- Day Spas listed in *COLOR* and *LARGER TYPE* have applied for and received accreditation by The Day Spa Association.
- Spa members marked with ✈ 'Year' are proud recipients of the "Distringuished Day Spa of the Year Award."

MIDWEST (continued)

SPA NAME	ADDRESS	PHONE/FAX	EMAIL/WEBSITE	DAY SPA	SALON w/SPA SERVICES	WELLNESS CENTER	AFFILIATED w/HEALTH CLUB	AFFILIATED w/MEDICAL FACILITY	SPA RESORT/DESTINATION	LIFESTYLE STORE	SPA RESTAURANT
Charlotte's Day Spa & Salon	20300 Chagrin Blvd. Shaker Heights, OH 44122	216-283-2400 f: 216-491-8666	Gen-Char@Stratos.net **charlottedayspa.com**	•	•						•
Davida Salon & Spa	28699 Chagrin Blvd. Woodmere Village, OH 44122	216-464-4722 f: 216-464-1450	CP358@aol.com **davidasalon.com**		•						
MARIO'S INTERNATIONAL SPA & HOTELS ✈2000	49 E. Garfield Rd. Aurora, OH 44202	330-562-9171 f: 330-562-5380	info@Marios-spa.com **marios-spa.com**	•	•	•	•	•	•	•	•
SASTUN SALON & DAY SPA	33705 Station St. Solon, OH 44139	440-349-0097 f: 440-349-2997	sastun@earthlink.net **members.Tripod.com/Sastun**								
Shear Design Salon & Day Spa	1215 Fourth St. N.W. New Philadelphia, OH 44663	330-364-2511 f: 330-343-5860	sdesign@tusco.net		•						
The Spa at Glenmoor	4191 Glenmoor Rd. N.W. Canton, OH 44718	330-966-3524 f: 330-498-4621	sgelb@glenmoorcc.com **glenmoor.cc.com**						•	•	
Vickie Lynn's Salon & Day Spa	4733 Hills & Dales Rd. Canton, OH 44708	330-479-1993 f: 330-479-1909	vickielynn@sssnet.com	•							
Toni's Salon & Spa	905 Second St. Wausau, WI 54403	715-842-2119	ToniToney@aol.com **tonishairdesign.com**	•							

SOUTHWEST

SPA NAME	ADDRESS	PHONE/FAX	EMAIL/WEBSITE	DAY SPA	SALON w/SPA SERVICES	WELLNESS CENTER	AFFILIATED w/HEALTH CLUB	AFFILIATED w/MEDICAL FACILITY	SPA RESORT/DESTINATION	LIFESTYLE STORE	SPA RESTAURANT
Elizabeth Arden Red Door Salon & Spas	3822 E. University Dr., No. 5 Phoenix, AZ 85034	800-59 ARDEN f: 800-57 ARDEN	**reddoorsalons.com**	•	•						
Par Exsalonce Salon and Day Spa	9160 E. Shea Blvd., Ste.106 Scottsdale, AZ 85260	480-860-0717 f: 480-860-6914		•							
Spa Du Soleil	7040 E. Third Ave. Scottsdale, AZ 85251	480-994-5400 f: 480-994-0591		•							
The Spa at Gainey Village	7477 E. Doubletree Ranch Rd. Scottsdale, AZ 85258	480-609-6980 f: 480-609-7999		•		•	•	•			
The Spa at Marriott Camelback Inn	5402 E. Lincoln Dr. Scottsdale, AZ 85253	800-92-CAMEL f: 480-596-7018	**camelbackinn.com**							•	•
THE STRESS LESS STEP	5115 N. Scottsdale Rd. Scottsdale, AZ 85250	800-794-7066 f: 480-945-1579	stresslessstep@aol.com **stresslessstep.com**	•		•					
The Sterling Institute	513 Camino De Los Marquez, Ste. D Santa Fe, NM 87501	505-984-3223 f: 505-988-5644	Murban@compuserve.com **thesterlinginstitute.com**			•					
Bodyworks	6201 Colleyville Blvd., Ste. 200 Colleyville, TX 76034	817-416-0715	**body-works.net**	•							
Daya	3208 Guadalupe Austin, TX 78705	512-374-1010 f: 512-452-6814	info@dayaenergy.com **dayaenergy.com**	•							
Eclipse Salon & Day Spa	904 S. Main St. Weatherford, TX 76086	817-341-0833 f: 817-599-3233	giggiedobbs@yahoo.com **eclipse-salon.com**		•						
Millennium Day Spa	1100 Lakeway Dr., Ste. 100 Austin, TX 78734	877-307-6772 f: 512-261-1724	info@millenniumdayspa.com **millenniumdayspa.com**	•							
Paulette's Day Spa	2171 Gilmen Rd. Longview, TX 75604	903-295-8090 f: 903-295-8091		•	•						
Serenity Day Spa	204 E. Austin Fredericksburg, TX 78624	830-990-1126 f: 830-990-2772	DSPAretreat@hotmail.com **serenitydSpa.com**	•							
The Greenhouse - Dallas	5560 W. Lovers Ln. Dallas, TX 75209	214-654-9800 f: 214-654-9807	**thegreenhousespa.com**	•							
The Greenhouse - Houston	2535 Kirby Dr. Houston, TX 77019	713-529-2444 f: 713-529-4557	**thegreenhousespa.com**	•							
The Woodhouse Day Spa	203 E. Stayton Victoria, TX 77901	361-572-8488 f: 361-570-7301	jenibishop@yahoo.com	•							
With Class - A Day Spa	621B Chase Dr. Tyler, TX 75701	903-581-1745 f: 903-581-1752		•							

ROCKY MOUNTAIN STATES

SPA NAME	ADDRESS	PHONE/FAX	EMAIL/WEBSITE	DAY SPA	SALON w/SPA SERVICES	WELLNESS CENTER	AFFILIATED w/HEALTH CLUB	AFFILIATED w/MEDICAL FACILITY	SPA RESORT/DESTINATION	LIFESTYLE STORE	SPA RESTAURANT
A+ European Body and Health	1510 Glen Ayr Dr., Ste. 11 Lakewood, CO 80215	303-233-0712 f: 303-233-0712	massage@a-eurobody-health.com **a-eurobody-health.com**	•							
City Spa Escapes	1630 Welton St., Ste. 300 Denver, CO 80202	303-623-0112 f: 303-892-5628	CitySpaEscapes@aol.com								
The Greenhouse - Denver	242 Milwaukee St. Denver, CO 80206	303-388-3800 f: 303-388-8807	**thegreenhousespa.com**	•							
Body Express	450 South Buffalo, Ste. 113 Las Vegas, NV 89145	702-804-0888 f: 702-804-0880		•							
Dolphin Court Salon & Day Spa	3455 South Durango Dr. Las Vegas, NV 89117	702-949-9999 f: 702-947-6006	info@dolphincourt.com **dolphincourt.com**	•	•						
On Site Stress Relief	c/o Excalibur Hotel & Casino 3850 Las Vegas Blvd. South Las Vegas, NV 89119	702-381-4529	geoshimo@earthlink.com								

Spa services comparison chart — column headers (listed top to bottom):

1. MASSAGES
2. CRANIAL MASSAGE
3. REIKI / SHIATSU
4. LA STONE / HOT STONE
5. LYMPH DRAINAGE
6. PREGNANCY TREATMENTS
7. REFLEXOLOGY
8. POLARITY
9. FACIALS
10. NON-SURGICAL FACE LIFT
11. MICRODERMABRASION
12. CHEMICAL PEELS
13. BODY PACKS / HERBAL WRAPS
14. BODY TONING / CONTOURING
15. EXFOLIATION
16. CELLULITE
17. ENDERMOLOGY
18. ARYURVEDA
19. HEAT TREATMENTS
20. AROMATHERAPY
21. HYDROTHERAPY / VICHY SHOWER
22. ACUPUNCTURE
23. OXYGEN THERAPY
24. ELECTROLYSIS
25. LASER HAIR REMOVAL
26. WAXING / SUGARING
27. MAKEUP CONSULTATION
28. PERMANENT MAKEUP
29. SPA MANICURE / PEDICURE
30. SCALP TREATMENTS
31. SPA HAIR CARE
32. PLASTIC SURGEON
33. DERMATOLOGIST
34. CHIROPRACTIC
35. HOMEOPATHIC OTHER
36. WEIGHT MANAGEMENT
37. NUTRITIONIST
38. FITNESS CLASSES
39. FITNESS EQUIPMENT
40. PERSONAL TRAINERS
41. YOGA / MEDITATION
42. LECTURES / WORKSHOPS
43. BODY / BATH / HAIR / SKIN
44. AROMATHERAPY
45. COSMETICS
46. SPA CLOTHING
47. GIFT CERTIFICATES
48. GIFT ITEMS
49. NUTRITIONAL SUPPLEMENTS
50. A-LA-CARTE SERVICES
51. PACKAGES
52. BRIDAL PACKAGES
53. MEN SPECIFIC TREATMENTS
54. FENG SHUI TESTED SPACE
55. STEAM / SAUNA
56. LOCKER ROOM
57. LOCKER ROOMS FOR MEN
58. PVT. TREATMENT ROOMS
59. MEETING / PARTY ROOM
60. PARKING
61. ACCOMMODATIONS NEARBY

SPA MEMBER DIRECTORY 2002

Type of Spa · **Salon Services** · **Retail**
Spa Treatments · **Medical Affiliation** · **Other**
Beauty Services · **Programs**

- Day Spas listed in *COLOR* and *LARGER TYPE* have applied for and received accreditation by The Day Spa Association.
- Spa members marked with →'Year' are proud recipients of the "Distringuished Day Spa of the Year Award."

SPA NAME	ADDRESS	PHONE/FAX	EMAIL/WEBSITE	DAY SPA	SALON w/SPA SERVICES	WELLNESS CENTER	AFFILIATED w/HEALTH CLUB	AFFILIATED w/MEDICAL FACILITY	SPA RESORT/DESTINATION	LIFESTYLE STORE	SPA RESTAURANT
NORTHWEST											
Solavie Spa & Salon	111 Washington Ave. / Ketchum, ID 83340	208-726-7211 / f: 208-726-7205	Sunvalleyspa@solavie.com / **solavie.com**	●	●	●				●	●
The Atrium Day Spa	51 Water St., Ste. 111 / Ashland, OR 97520	541-488-4088 / f: 541-488-8692	info@atriumdayspa.com / **atriumdayspa.com**	●							
The Pointe at Hawthorn Farm Athletic Club	4800 N.E. Beiknap Ct. / Hillsboro, OR 97124	503-640-6404 / f: 503-640-0644	pointe@hawthornfarmathletic.com / **hawthornfarmathletic.com**				●				
Essence Day Spa	371 N. 200 West / Bountiful, UT 84010	801-294-7534	EssenceDaySpa@cs.com	●	●						
Gene Juarez Grand Salon & Spa	550 106th N.E., No. 105 / Bellevue, WA 98004	425-455-5511	**genejuarez.com**	●	●						
Gene Juarez Grand Salon & Spa	6th & Pine, 4th Fl. / Seattle, WA 98101	206-326-6000	**genejuarez.com**	●	●						
Gene Juarez Salon & Spa	16449 N.E. 74th St. / Redmond Town Center / Redmond, WA 98052	425-882-9000	**genejuarez.com**	●	●						
Gene Juarez Salon & Spa	1070 Southcenter Mall / Seattle, WA 98188	206-431-8888	**genejuarez.com**	●	●						
Gene Juarez Salon & Spa	1139 Tacoma Mall / Tacoma, WA 98409	253-472-9999	**genejuarez.com**	●	●						
Kathleen's Salon & Day Spa	22021 Old Owen Rd. / Monroe, WA 98272	360-794-3395 / f: 425-788-0903	Kathleen@Premier1.net / **superpages.com/kathleensbeautyanddayspa**		●						
Sherwood Hills Resort & Spa (under development)	Hwy. 89-91, Sardine Canyon / Wellsville, UT 84339	435-245-5054 / 435-245-4183	rmkinut@aol.com / **sherwoodhillsresort.com**					●			
The Hide Away Spa	606 E. Morris St., P.O. Box 427 / LaConner, WA 98257	360-466-0289		●							
Watersedge Health Club & Spa	911 O Ave. / Anacortes, WA 98221	360-299-2180	akj@ewjlaw.com					●			
ALASKA											
Body Essentials Massage & Day Spa	2055 Jordan Ave. / Juneau, AK 99801	877-789-5900 / f: 907-789-5537	bodyessentials@juneaualaska.com	●							
Karlene's Lotus Day Spa	43335 K-Beach Rd., No. 8 / Soldotna, AK 99669	907-262-7977	karlene@ptialaska.net	●							
HAWAII											
Na Ho'ola Spa (Hyatt Regency Waikiki Resort & Spa)	2424 Kalakaua Ave. / Honolulu, HI 96815	808-921-6097 / f: 808-924-3409	afukui@hyattwaikiki.com / **hyatt.com**						●		
Paul Brown Salon Day Spa	1200 Ala Moana Blvd. / Honolulu, HI 96814	808-591-1881 / f: 808-596-0755	pbsalon@aol.com / **paulbrownhawaii.com**	●	●						
Indulgence Salon	99-165 Moanalua Rd., No. 302 / Aiea, HI 96701	808-487-1981		●							
CANADA											
Bodyworks Salon & Day Spa	1702 Bow Valley Trl. / Canmore, ALB T1W 1N5 CANADA	403-678-5746 / f: 403-678-5646	Bdywkspa@telusplanet.net	●	●						
Elm Hurst Inn	P.O. Box 123 / Ingersoll, ON N5C 3K1 CANADA	519-485-5521 / f: 519-485-6579	pat@elmhurstinn.com / **elmhurstinn.com**						●		
Images International Salon & Spa	280 N. Service Rd. / Oakville, ON L6M 2S2 CANADA	905-338-3333 / f: 905-849-7544	images2@on.ailon.com / **thespratimages.com**		●						
Spa at the Mill	8 Cataraqui St. / Kingston, ON K7K 1Z7 CANADA	514-544-1166 / f: 613-544-7654	information@spaatthemill.com / **spaatthemill.com**	●							
FAYEZ BEAUTY SPA →2000 2001	2224 Wharncliffe Rd. South / London, ON N6P 1L1 CANADA	519-652-2780 / f: 519-652-9603	visitus@fayezbeautyspa.com / **fayezbeautyspa.com**	●	●						
My Sanctuary Spa	218 Carlton St. / Toronto, ON M5A 2L1 CANADA	416-966-4772 / f: 416-922-4772	mysanctuaryspa@home.com / **mysanctuaryspa.com**	●							
Orient Retreat (Danger Figure Enterprises)	3330 Midland Ave., Unit 28 / Scarborough, ON M1V 5E7 CANADA	416-754-7389 / f: 416-754-1397	canada@enjoyspa.com / **enjoyspa.com**	●						●	●
Nefertiti Spa	180 Steeles Ave., Unit 17 / Thornhill, ON L4J 2L1 CANADA	905-886-8587 / 905-886-1662	inga@nefertiti-spa.ca / **nerfertiti-spa.ca**	●							
Dianne Mauch Esthetics & Day Spa	283B Park Ave. / Thunder Bay, ON P7B 1C4 CANADA	807-345-5484	Dianemauch@baynet.net	●							
The Village Spa Ltd.	2901 Bayview Ave. / Toronto, ON M2K 1E6 CANADA	416-224-1101 / f: 416-224-8969	**toronto.com/thevillagespa**	●							
Estetica Beauty Institute	2407 Dougall Ave. / Windsor, ON N8X 1T3 CANADA	519-969-9848 / f: 519-969-6332	info@estetica.com / **estetica.com**	●							
Institut de Beauté Carol St.Pierre Salon & Spa	33 Wharf Rd., P.O. Box 848 / Hudson, QP J0P 1H0 CANADA	450-458-5607 / f: 450-455-5534	institutcsp@securenet.net / **carolest-pierre.com**	●							

CRANIAL MASSAGE | REIKI / SHIATSU | LA STONE / HOT STONE | LYMPH DRAINAGE | PREGNANCY TREATMENTS | REFLEXOLOGY | POLARITY | FACIALS | NON-SURGICAL FACE LIFT | MICRODERMABRASION | CHEMICAL PEELS | BODY PACKS / HERBAL WRAPS | BODY TONING / CONTOURING | EXFOLIATION | CELLULITE | ENDERMOLOGY | ARYURVEDA | HEAT TREATMENTS | AROMATHERAPY | HYDROTHERAPY / VICHY SHOWER | ACUPUNCTURE | OXYGEN THERAPY | ELECTROLYSIS | LASER HAIR REMOVAL | WAXING / SUGARING | MAKEUP CONSULTATION | PERMANENT MAKEUP | SPA MANICURE / PEDICURE | SCALP TREATMENTS | SPA HAIR CARE | PLASTIC SURGEON | DERMATOLOGIST | CHIROPRACTIC | HOMEOPATHIC OTHER | WEIGHT MANAGEMENT | NUTRITIONIST | FITNESS CLASSES | FITNESS EQUIPMENT | PERSONAL TRAINERS | YOGA / MEDITATION | LECTURES / WORKSHOPS | BODY / BATH / HAIR / SKIN | AROMATHERAPY | COSMETICS | SPA CLOTHING | GIFT CERTIFICATES | GIFT ITEMS | NUTRITIONAL SUPPLEMENTS | A-LA-CARTE SERVICES | PACKAGES | BRIDAL PACKAGES | MEN SPECIFIC TREATMENTS | FENG SHUI TESTED SPACE | STEAM / SAUNA | LOCKER ROOM | LOCKER ROOMS FOR MEN | PVT. TREATMENT ROOMS | MEETING / PARTY ROOM | PARKING | ACCOMMODATIONS NEARBY

SPA MEMBER DIRECTORY 2002

	Type of Spa		Salon Services		Retail
	Spa Treatments		Medical Affiliation		Other
	Beauty Services		Programs		

- Day Spas listed in *COLOR* and *LARGER TYPE* have applied for and received accreditation by The Day Spa Association.
- Spa members marked with 'Year' are proud recipients of the "Distringuished Day Spa of the Year Award."

SPA NAME	ADDRESS	PHONE/FAX	EMAIL/WEBSITE	DAY SPA	SALON w/SPA SERVICES	WELLNESS CENTER	AFFILIATED w/HEALTH CLUB	AFFILIATED w/MEDICAL FACILITY	SPA RESORT/DESTINATION	LIFESTYLE STORE
MIDWEST (continued)										
Joie De Vivre	P.O. Box 1402 Yellowknife, NT X1A 2P1 CANADA	867-873-2123 f: 867-920-2398	**ajcip@internorth.com**	•		•	•			
MEXICO										
Paradise Village Beach Resort & Spa	Ave. Cocoteros, No. 001 Nuevo Vallarta, Nay. 63731 MEXICO	0-11-52-322-66727 f: 322-667263	spa@paradisevillage.com **paradisevillage.com**						•	
Neways Healing Center & Day Spa	Ave. Paseo de las Garzas 510 N. Hotel Zone Puerto Vallarta, Jalisco MEXICO	0-11-52-322-52593 f: 0-11-52-322-50590	ana4neways@yahoo.com	•		•				•
Elizabeth Ontiveros (under development)	Cipres, No. 4605, Valles de la Silla Guadalupe, N.L. 67180 MEXICO	0-11-52-83-614909								
CENTRAL/SOUTH AMERICA										
Soulshine Resort & Spa	1 Placencia Point Placencia BELIZE	501-623 347 f: 501-623 369	spa@soulshine.com **soulshine.com**	•					•	
Sao Paulo Day Spa Health Care	R. Viscon de Nacar, No.147, Real Parque Sao Paulo 05685-010 BRAZIL	0-11-55-11-3758-9222 f: 0-11-55-11-3051-3377	dayspa@dayspa.com.br **dayspa.com.br**	•	•	•	•	•		
Nora Castro	Cardenal Belarmino JO82 Vitacura, Santiago CHILE	0-11-56-2-211-5006 f: 0-11-56-2-211 5006	norita_clyahoo.es							
Purguey Spa	Ed. Faruenca Calle 8 - La Urbina Caracas, Miranda VENEZUELA	0-11-58-02-241 3345 f: 0-11-58-02 2427740								
ASIA										
Institut Esthétique de Suisse Limited	Chinachem Century Tower, 33rd Fl. 178 Gloucester Rd. Wanchai HONG KONG	0-11-852-2803 4768 f: 0-11-852-2803 4628	edes_asia@esthedes.com Edes-spa.com	•		•	•			
Esthétique de Suisse Beauty Spa	Level 24-2 (Penthouse) Menara Genesis No. 33 Jalan Sultan Ismail 50250 Kuala Lumpur MALAYSIA	0-11-603-241 2845 f: 0-11-603-242 1277	edes@tm.net.my	•		•	•			
Esthétique de Suisse Beauty Spa	Hyatt Regency Hotel J.B. Johor Bahru MALAYSIA			•		•	•			
Danger Figure Spa	4th Fl., No. 10, Ln. 209 An-Ho Rd.-Section 2 Taiwan 106 TAIPEI	0-11-080-000-816 f: 0-11-886-2-2739-8145	Taiwan@dangerfigure.com **dangerfigure.com**	•					•	•
MIDDLE EAST										
Physi Tech (under development)	7 Barazany St. Tel Aviv 69121 ISRAEL	972-3-642-8259 f: 972-3-642-7444	worldwide@lanteck.net						•	
EUROPE										
Secret Garden Aesthetic-Slimming-Alternative Therapies Day Spa	Bagdat Cad. San Ap., No. 304/18 Caddebostan, Istanbul 81080 TURKEY	0-11-90-216-385 64 52 f: 0-11-90-216-363 7182	secretgardens@ssaglikguzellik.com **saglikguzellik.com**	•	•	•	•			

MASSAGES | CRANIAL MASSAGE | REIKI / SHIATSU | LA STONE / HOT STONE | LYMPH DRAINAGE | PREGNANCY TREATMENTS | REFLEXOLOGY | POLARITY | FACIALS | NON-SURGICAL FACE LIFT | MICRODERMABRASION | CHEMICAL PEELS | BODY PACKS / HERBAL WRAPS | BODY TONING / CONTOURING | EXFOLIATION | CELLULITE | ENDERMOLOGY | ARYURVEDA | HEAT TREATMENTS | AROMATHERAPY | HYDROTHERAPY / VICHY SHOWER | ACUPUNCTURE | OXYGEN THERAPY | ELECTROLYSIS | LASER HAIR REMOVAL | WAXING / SUGARING | MAKEUP CONSULTATION | PERMANENT MAKEUP | SPA MANICURE / PEDICURE | SCALP TREATMENTS | SPA HAIR CARE | PLASTIC SURGEON | DERMATOLOGIST | CHIROPRACTIC | HOMEOPATHIC OTHER | WEIGHT MANAGEMENT | NUTRITIONIST | FITNESS CLASSES | FITNESS EQUIPMENT | PERSONAL TRAINERS | YOGA / MEDITATION | LECTURES / WORKSHOPS | BODY / BATH / HAIR / SKIN | AROMATHERAPY | COSMETICS | SPA CLOTHING | GIFT CERTIFICATES | GIFT ITEMS | NUTRITIONAL SUPPLEMENTS | A-LA-CARTE SERVICES | PACKAGES | BRIDAL PACKAGES | MEN SPECIFIC TREATMENTS | FENG SHUI TESTED SPACE | STEAM / SAUNA | LOCKER ROOM | LOCKER ROOMS FOR MEN | PVT. TREATMENT ROOMS | MEETING / PARTY ROOM | PARKING | ACCOMMODATIONS NEARBY

Procedure:

Cold Affusion, Right and Left Arm
Temperature: 65°F

Upper body is bent over the affusion rack (bathtub).

The client inhales and exhales evenly while the cold affusion begins on the back side of the right hand.

Hose up the outside of the arm to the shoulder. Stay in place, then move downwards inside the arm to the palm.

Switch to the left arm.

Repeat the procedure three to four times.

Wipe the water off with hands. Do not towel dry.

The affusion should be followed by active exercise or one hour of rest.

WATER AFFUSIONS

Arm Affusion—
Alternate Temperature

Indications: Fatigue, heart palpitations, cold hands, low blood pressure

Contraindications: Coronary heart ailments, asthma

Effects: Refreshing, stimulates blood circulation

Equipment: Shower hose

Procedure:

1. **Warm Affusion, Right and Left Arm**
   Temperature: 97–100°F

   Upper body is bent over the affusion rack.

   Start on the back side of the right hand. Move up the outside of the arm to the shoulder.

   Maintain position until the client feels warm and a light redness appears.

   Continue to hose downwards inside the arm to the palms.

   Repeat on the left arm.

2. **Cold Affusion, Right and Left Arm**
   Temperature: 65°F

   Start on the back side of the right hand, and hose up the outside of the arm to the shoulder.
   Maintain hose position.

   Continue down inside the right arm to the palm of the hand.

   Repeat the same stroke on the left arm.

3. Repeat Warm Affusion.

4. Repeat Cold Affusion.

5. Wipe the water off with hands. Do not towel dry.

   The affusion should be followed by active exercise or one hour of bed rest.

Face Affusion—
Cold Temperature

Indications: Fatigue, headache, migraine

Contraindications: Glaucoma (eye ailments or disorders), acute sinusitis

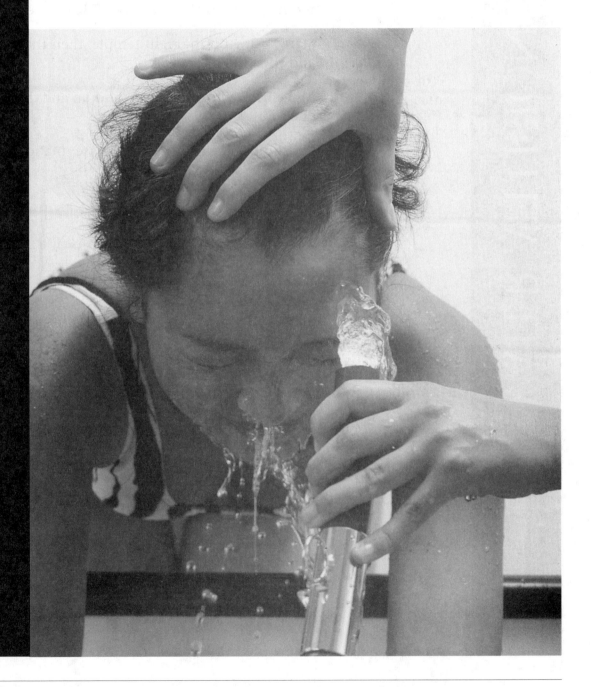

Effects:	Refreshes, stimulates blood circulation, reduces wrinkles
Equipment:	Shower hose
Temperature:	65°F
Procedure:	Place towel around neck.

Throughout the affusion, the client should inhale through the mouth. If necessary, interrupt hosing momentarily so client can catch his or her breath.

Start hosing on the right temple, then the forehead, and then the left temple.

Move back across forehead, and up and down the left cheek.

Finish hosing with three clockwise rotations.

Dry face with a towel.

NOTE

The cold face affusion can be done more than once a day.

Chest Affusion— Cold Temperature

Indications: Weak immune system, overall fatigue

Contraindications: Asthma, oversensitivity to cold

Effects: Increases metabolic rate, refreshes, increases tissue elasticity through increased blood circulation

Equipment: $3/4$ inch hose, $3^1/2$ feet long

Procedure: Upper body is bent over affusion rack.

Start hosing on the right hand, moving up the outside of the arm to the shoulder.

Continue to hose shoulder until a light redness appears.

Hose down inside of the arm to the hand.

Repeat the same stroke on the left side.

Move the hose inside the left arm up to the armpit again, crossing back over the chest twice.

Then hose the chest in a figure eight, moving back to the armpit, down the inside of the arm, to the hand.

Wipe off the water with hands. Do not towel dry.

The affusion should be followed by active exercise or one hour of bed rest.

Chest Affusion—
Alternate Temperature

Indications: Weak immune system, fatigue, low blood pressure, cold hands, oversensitivity to cold

Contraindications: Coronary heart ailments, asthma

Effects: Increases metabolic rate, refreshes, stimulates blood circulation and blood flow

Equipment: 3/4 inch hose, 3 1/2 feet long

Procedure:

1. Warm Affusion
Temperature: 97–100°F

Upper body is bent over affusion rack.

Start hosing on back side of the right hand, and move up the outside of the arm to the shoulder. Maintain hose position until client feels warm and the skin appears red.

Then hose down the inside of the arm to the hand.

Repeat the same stroke on the left side.

Then go up inside the left arm to the armpit, crossing back over the chest twice.

Hose the chest in a figure eight pattern.

Move back to the armpit, and down the inside of the arm to the hand.

2. Cold Affusion
Temperature: 97–100°F

Repeat the procedure using cold water. The cold affusion should be done more quickly than the warm one.

3. Repeat warm affusion.

4. Repeat cold affusion.

5. Wipe off the water with hands. Do not towel dry.

Exercise or one hour rest should follow the affusion.

WATER AFFUSIONS

Lumbar Affusion—
Increasing Temperature

Indications: Acute lumbago, sciatica, spinal musculature tension

Contraindications: Acute low back disorders

Effects: Hyperemia, increases blood flow, relaxes lower back muscles, reduces lower back spasm, reduces tension in the abdominal and pelvic region

Equipment: Shower hose, comfortable chair

Procedure: Client sits on a chair or on the side of a tub.

Start hosing the lower back. The water temperature should start at 93°F and gradually be increased to 109°F.

The treatment is finished when the skin is noticeably red.

Dry with a towel.

Following lumbar affusion with one hour of rest is recommended.

> **NOTE**
> The temperature must increase gradually.

Neck Affusion—
Increasing Temperature

Indications: Cervical muscle tension, migraine headaches

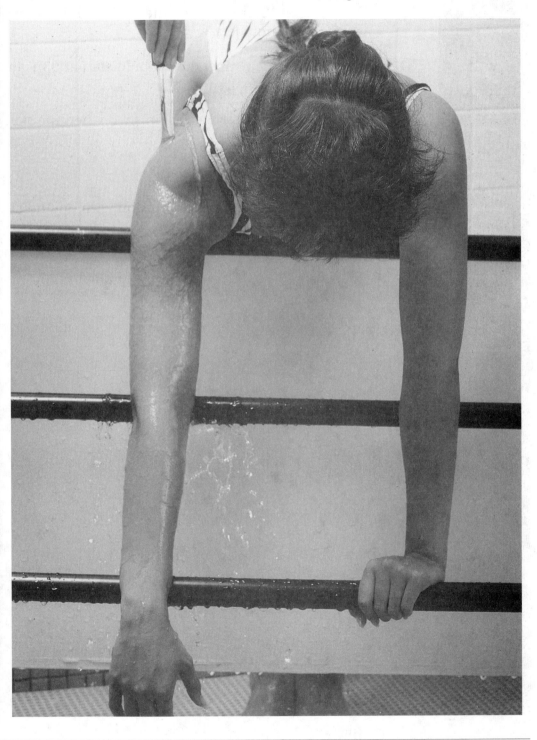

Contraindications: Glaucoma, high blood pressure, cardiac insufficiency

Effects: Muscular relaxation, increased blood circulation

Equipment: Shower hose

Procedure: Upper body is bent over the affusion rack.

Water runs over the neck and down the left and right shoulders.

The temperature should start at 93°F and be increased gradually to 109°F.

The treatment is finished when the skin is noticeably red.

Dry with a towel.

Following neck affusion with one hour of rest is recommended.

> **NOTE**
>
> The temperature must increase gradually.

CHAPTER 9

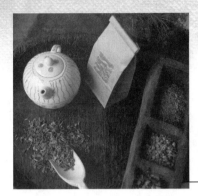

AFFUSIONS UNDER PRESSURE

Scotch Hose Shower Blitz Jet Affusion

Affusions under pressure have a strong mechanical effect along with the thermal effect. They are administered from a hose with a nozzle, which narrows the stream of water to about five millimeters. The affusion under pressure is administered from a distance of three meters. The temperature is usually cold, as for simple affusions, but it can also be hot or alternately cold and hot.

Kneipp affusions are an excellent vascular exercise for the athlete, and they also help produce a general toughening and reviving effect on the entire body. The influence of the cold water—50° to 59°F—creates a hyperemia. Cold affusions are particularly effective following extreme exertions, especially in warm weather with accompanying heat buildup. They are effective both in the breaks between individual events in sports involving several separate competitions and during endurance events.

As an approximate guide to the pressure force, hold the nozzle of the hose horizontally thirty inches above the floor. The stream of water should hit the floor about eighteen feet away.

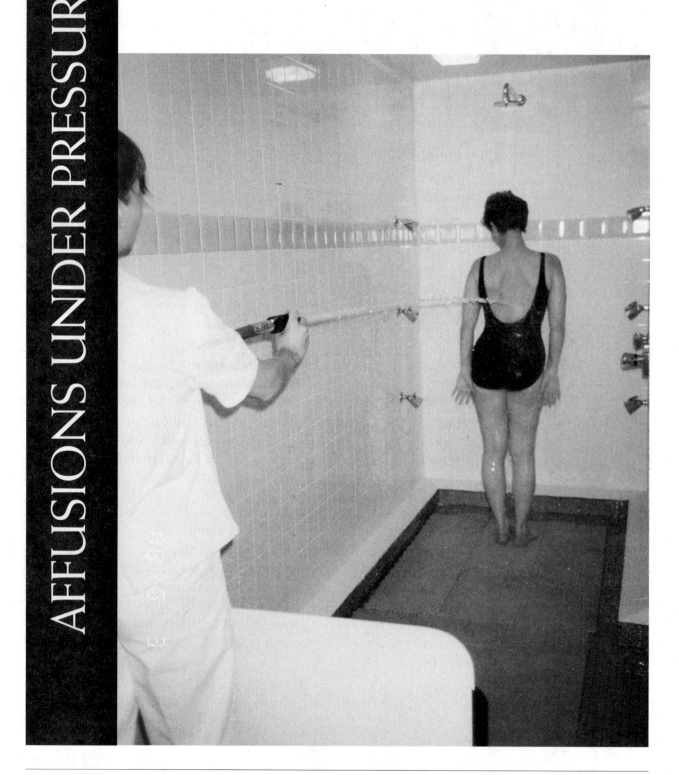

AFFUSIONS UNDER PRESSURE

Scotch Hose Shower Blitz Jet Affusion–Hot Temperature

Indications: Arthritis in non-inflammatory stage, chronic lumbago, muscular tension, irregular menstruation cycle, mild blood circulation problems

Contraindications: Nervosity, varicose veins, inelasticity of the skin, heart or blood circulation problems, any inflammation

Effects: Increases metabolic rate, improves the immune system

Equipment: Hose with jet nozzle

Temperature: 104–113°F

Procedure: The treatment begins with a temperate spray, produced by pressing the fingertips into the jet at the nozzle.

The treatment lasts for two to three minutes and is concluded with a full body spray at a moderate temperature.

Example of a Kneipp Hydro-Herbal Spa Treatment Sequence

The Five B's to Stress Reduction

1.	Bath, herbal	10 minutes
2.	Blitz-jet affusion, hot temperature	2–3 minutes
3.	Bath, herbal	5 minutes
4.	Blitz-jet affusion, hot temperature	2–3 minutes
5.	Bed rest	1 hour

Duration: Total treatment time approximately two hours

Procedure: The blitz-jet affusion and herbal bath routine has the following sequence:

Assist client into a 97°F herbal bath (pine needle, hay flower).

After ten minutes, follow with a hot blitz-jet affusion lasting two to three minutes.

Follow with a second hot herbal bath for five minutes.

Follow with another two to three minute hot blitz-jet affusion.

The body temperature is reduced with a moderate temperature spray shower.

Finish with an hour of bed rest.

NOTE

It is imperative that the client rest for at least one hour.

CHAPTER 10

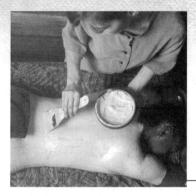

SHOWERS AND STEAM SHOWERS

Showers include all applications of water or steam that are administered under pressure. Showers are divided into cold, neutral, warm, and hot. Hot showers and extended showers are preferred for rheumatic disorders. Showers can be rain or fan, with a gentle low pressure stream or jet, or a direct powerful pressure, and are used in various temperatures.

For the athlete, warm showers after training or competition have a generally loosening and relaxing effect, in addition to being cleansing. Cold showers have a tonic effect on the blood vessels and are a good way to conclude a warm shower. Steam showers can be used to improve muscular recovery after competition. The steam shower is also suited for the treatment of residual damage, such as occurs in contractures, scars, and rheumatic disorders.

In a steam shower, the steam is sprayed onto the skin at a mild comfortable pressure and a temperature of about 110°F. The treating person should keep a distance of six feet from the client, as the steam can otherwise scald.

Cold Shower

Definition: The shower is used as cold as, and as long as, the client can tolerate it. The endurance to cold will increase as the procedure is prolonged.

Contraindications: Cardiovascular instability

Effects: Overcomes fatigue, tonic effect, reduces elevated body temperature

Hot Shower

Definition: A light spray–rain shower for two to five minutes with temperature from 100°F to 104°F eases neuralgic pain and comforts the body.

Contraindications: Any form of swelling, lymph edema

Effects: Prepares client for a cold treatment, alleviates pain, soothes irritated skin

Neutral Shower

A light gentle-spray shower for four to six minutes in lukewarm (92–97°F), body-temperature water relaxes the body by contracting the circulatory blood system. The reaction is similar to that with a long neutral bath.

Alternate Hot and Cold Shower

Always begin with the hot shower and do not shock the body. The alternating temperature has the most body hardening and conditioning effect. Equal amounts of hot and cold water or unequal amounts can be applied with emphasis on the hot water.

Swiss Shower

Definition:

This cascading vertical body spray shower has nine or more sprays. It creates a gentle or vigorous rain shower from the ankles to the shoulders from above. It is commonly used before and/or after an herbal body wrap, skin exfoliation, and massage therapy.

The treatment provides relief from symptoms of tension, insomnia, and stress. A true shower treatment is actually a full body alternating-temperature hydro-massage performed by the effect of the shower heads.

Indications:

Chronic back pain, insomnia, vascular instability

Contraindications:

Cardiovascular insufficiencies, venous disorders, thromboses, varices

Temperature:

103°F to 70°F, to 103°F to 65°F, and so on

> **NOTE**
> Using the Vichy shower procedure to do a salt glow exfoliation, keep a warm water hose on the client's abdomen.

Vichy Shower

Definition:

The Vichy shower therapy was originally created for clients with apoplexy, paraplegia, quadriplegia, and cardiovascular insufficiencies. The Vichy shower is a

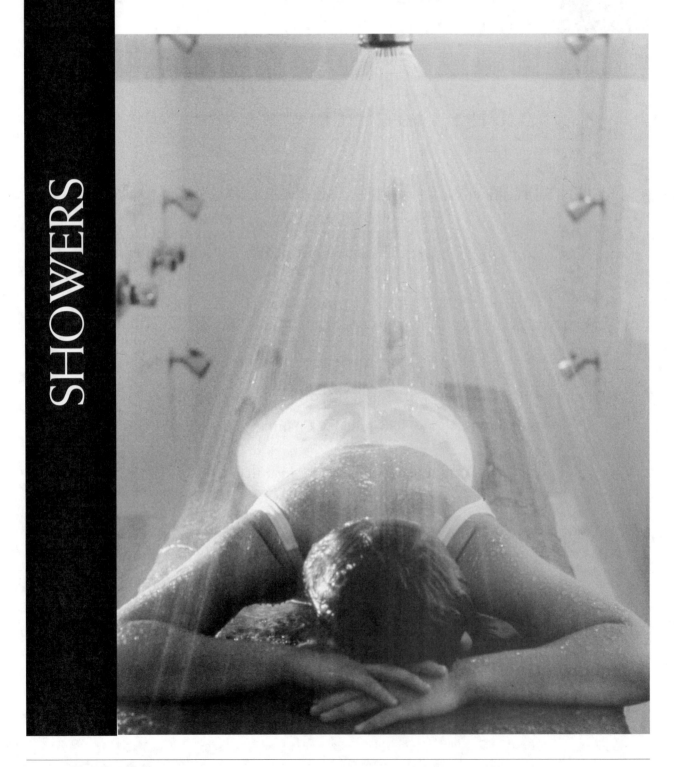

horizontal shower bar with shower nozzles arranged so that the entire body, situated on a table, is covered with a gentle water stream.

The Vichy shower therapy is a form of hydromassage with a temperature of about 105°F or contrast temperature (warm-cool) application.

For optimal vascular results, the client is brushed with a soft bristle brush.

Indications:	Chronic fatigue, mild hypertension, lymphatic congestion, skin exfoliation, and cleansing
Contraindications:	Vascular instability, open skin ailments, lymph edema, pregnancy

SHOWERS

CHAPTER 11

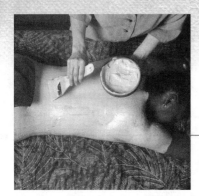

KNEIPP ABLUTION

Washing Down with a Wet Cloth or Mitten

KNEIPP ABLUTION

Definition:

Ablution, performed with a wet cloth, is the mildest form of Kneipp water application. Ablution differs from usual cleansing procedures. The washing procedure is divided into whole and partial body washings. Treatment should take place in a draft-free, warm room. A coarse linen wash cloth is recommended for the procedure. Water should be applied evenly to the body parts being washed. The stimulating effect of the washing (especially on the skin's circulation) may be augmented with the addition of vinegar to the water. Use one part vinegar to two parts water.

Effects:

Enhances blood circulation, relaxes, activates the production of heat in the body. The toxic substances in the blood will be increasingly eliminated and even prevented in the limbs.

WARNING

The fundamental rule to be strictly observed without exceptions is applicable to all water treatments: Anyone whose body is not sufficiently warm, or who is shivering, should not receive any cold water applications.

Ablution, Washing of Upper Extremities, Chest, and Back

Indications: Stress syndrome, dysfunctional thermo-regulatory system, rheumatism, colds, fever

Contraindications: Oversensitivity to cold

Effect: Toughens the skin, improves circulation, stimulates metabolism

Equipment: Coarse linen washcloth

Procedure: Dip a coarse linen washcloth in cold water.

Wash the right arm—first the exterior, from the shoulder to the hand, then the interior to the armpit.

Move to left arm—same procedure.

Stroke across the chest and then clockwise across the abdomen.

The back side is rubbed down with several strokes.

Ablution should be performed as quickly as possible.

Do not dry. Have client dress in pajamas and assist him or her into a warm bed.

Water additives: Vinegar

Ablution, Washing of Lower Extremities, Buttocks

Indications: Stress syndrome, dysfunction of the body's thermoregulatory system (rheumatism, cold, fever), poor circulation, insomnia, varicose veins, thyroid overactivity

Contraindications: Oversensitivity to cold, bladder or kidney infection, inflammation or infection of the female pelvic organs

Effects: Toughens skin, reduces insomnia, stimulates metabolism, promotes digestive process

Equipment: Coarse linen washcloth, cold water

Procedure: Dip a coarse linen washcloth into cold water.

Wash the right leg—first exterior front.

Move to the left leg front.

Then wash the right leg back.

Move to the left leg back.

End with the soles of the feet.

Ablution should be performed as quickly as possible.

Do not dry.

Have client dress in either a nightdress or pajamas and get into a warm bed.

Water additives: Vinegar

Ablution, Washing Down of the Whole Body

Indications: Immune deficiency, poor circulation, insomnia, chronic rheumatic disease

Contraindications: Oversensitivity to cold

Equipment: Coarse linen washcloth, cold water

Procedure: Dip a coarse linen washcloth into cold water.

Wash the right arm front—exterior then interior.

Move to the left arm front—exterior then interior.

Move to the throat, across chest, and then use clockwise strokes across abdomen.

Wash the right leg—front, start with foot.

Move to the left leg—front, start with foot.

Wash the back side down with several strokes.

Starting at the heel, wash the right leg back.

Wash the left leg back, again starting with the heel.

Wash the right and left soles of the feet.

Ablution should be performed as quickly as possible.

Do not dry.

Have client dress in either a nightdress or pajamas and cover him or her well in a warm bed.

> **NOTE**
>
> For bedridden clients, this is a good procedure for body hardening and conditioning.

Ablution, Washing Down of the Abdomen

KNEIPP ABLUTION

Indications:	Insomnia, dysfunction of the digestive organs
Contraindications:	Oversensitivity to cold, inflammation, bladder or kidney infection
Effects:	Alleviates insomnia, stimulates digestive organs
Equipment:	Coarse linen washcloth, cold water
Procedure:	Warm the bed before starting the treatment. Assist the client into a supine position on the bed. Bend the client's knees into a comfortable position.
	Dip coarse linen washcloth into cold water.
	Rub the abdomen with the washcloth clockwise twenty to forty times.
	Immerse washcloth several times during treatment.
	Allow client to rest after treatment.
Duration:	Two to five minutes
Water Additives:	Vinegar

Ablution, Washing Down of Arms and Legs

KNEIPP ABLUTION

Indications:	Fever, acute infections
Contraindications:	Oversensitivity to cold, cold hands or feet
Effects:	Reduces fever, increases perspiration, improves circulation, refreshes
Equipment:	Coarse linen washcloth, cold water
Procedure:	Assist client into bed, then dip a coarse washcloth into cold water.
	Washing down begins with lower part of the legs or lower part of the arms.
	Ablution should be performed as quickly as possible.
	Do not dry.
	Cover client well with a blanket.
	If the client feels warm again, repeat the procedure. The procedure can be repeated several times in an hour.
Water Additives:	Vinegar

CHAPTER 12

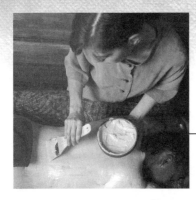

BODY WRAPS

Body wraps and body packs are ancient body treatments. Water and cloths have long been used to create and develop specific states in the body. Each step of these procedures should be followed cautiously.

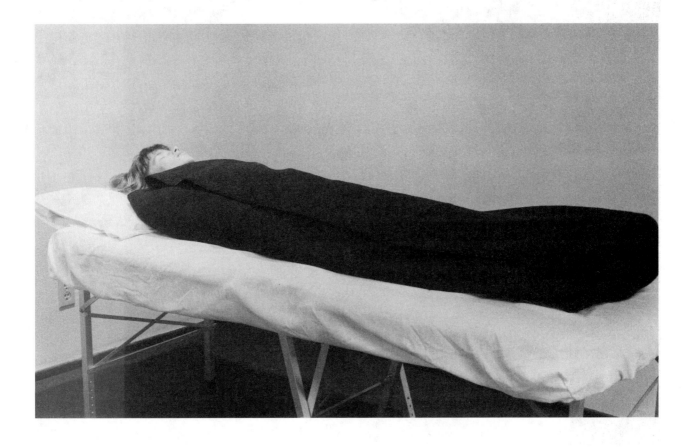

Dry Blanket Wrap

Definition: The dry blanket pack is Priessnitz's original preparation for creating perspiration and inducing the elimination of liquids. It is a valuable therapy for chronic rheumatism (the dry pack, unlike the hot moist pack, does not make you feel weak). This very simple wrapping produces a powerful reaction.

Indications: Chronic rheumatism

Contraindications: Fever, diabetes, arteriosclerosis, cardiac weakness

Effect: Induces perspiration

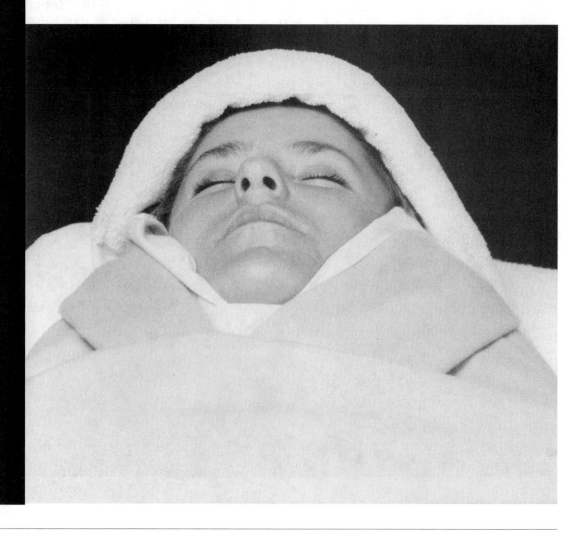

BODY WRAPS

Equipment: Linen sheets, wool blankets, large, coarse towel

Procedure: Prepare the table with two blankets, one on top of the other.

Prepare a hot water bottle. This is especially useful for a weak client, or one who will need a boost in heating the body.

Prepare a hot herbal tea: peppermint, thyme, sage, or red raspberry.

Assist client into hot bath or hot foot bath. Client should remain in bath fifteen to thirty minutes. Apply a cold compress to the forehead.

Tuck the blanket around the body. To increase perspiration, apply hot water bottles to the soles of the feet and the sides of the body.

Allow client to rest in a warm, well-ventilated room for thirty minutes. Apply a cold compress to the head.

Sponge the body with cold water, or immerse the entire body in a full cold bath for thirty seconds to one minute.

Vigorously dry the body with a large coarse towel, and allow the client to rest again.

Cool Moist Blanket Body Wrap

Definition:

This wrap is the most effective and powerful of all the water therapies. While the directions for this pack may seem complicated at first, it is actually only a long, double body compress in which the legs are separated by a layer of cloth. This wrap is exceptional in helping the client to overcome fevers, and a three-quarter or half pack may be used several times a day. It is also very helpful for most chronic diseases, and in detoxifying the body.

Indications:

Elevated body temperature, nervousness (for tonic or sedative wrap), oncoming cold or flu, skin ailments

Procedure:

Prepare a hot water bottle.

Prepare the table with protective material by laying two large blankets so that the ends are lower than the sides of the bed. Then place a large, dry white sheet on top of the blankets. (You will later lay a cold wet sheet on top of the dry sheet. See below.)

Have a perspiration-inducing drink, such as peppermint tea, ready.

Have containers of cold water for the cold compress ready.

Have hot water bottle ready (it will warm the client's feet).

Prepare the damp wet sheet by plunging a large white cotton sheet into cold water, and wringing it out so that it is damp and not too wet. Keep it in a sink, to either apply directly after the bath while client is standing or to place on the bed on the dry sheet when the client emerges from the bath.

Prepare a full hot bath or a hot foot bath. A full hot bath is preferred for total relaxation, sedation, and perspiration induction. You can increase the detoxification effect by adding up to five cups of mineral salts, a cup of essential pine oil, or a cup of essential meadow flower oil to the bathwater.

Apply a cold compress to client's forehead. Have client enter the hot water or take a hot foot bath. Furnish herbal drinks. The bath may last from fifteen to thirty minutes depending on comfort. Perspiration starts.

Assist client out of the bath.

The original classic wrap method is to place the wet sheet from the sink on the table before the client enters the bath. Wrap the client's body in large towels, discard the towels, and quickly help the client lie down on the bed on the cold damp sheet with arms raised. As rapidly as possible, bring the right half of the wet sheet over the trunk and right leg. Tuck it in, and lay the loose folds between the legs. Lower the arms. Bring the left half of the sheet over the front of body. Cover shoulders, trunk, arms, and left leg. Turn client on left side, and tuck the sheet under the right side. Tug the cotton sheet tightly so that no air can emerge. It should be snug, but not tight. Do not let two skin surfaces touch. The sheet is between the skin and the blanket. Fold the blankets snugly over the client's body in envelope fashion.

If the client feels weak, place a hot water bottle on feet to speed the warming-up reaction. Additional light covers may also be added to speed the reaction. They can be applied from chin to ankles, but do not cover feet. Tuck in around shoulders, and remove extra blankets as soon as the heat reaction occurs.

For a very anxious client who cannot bear the thought of being wrapped, use a less extensive wrap up to the armpits. The arms are left free.

End the application by washing the body with diluted vinegar (ablution). Do this in sections so that client does not chill.

Completely dry the skin.

Since this is a detoxifying perspiration-inducing technique, and is not energizing, client should rest and drink a lot of juice.

BODY WRAPS

Hot Moist Blanket Body Wrap

Definition: This linen wrap is applied in the same way as a damp sheet wrap except that the linen sheet or blanket (preferred) is dipped into hot water, 110°F. Wring dry, as the wet blanket loses heat very quickly. The value of the hot moist linen wrap is that it induces perspiration very quickly, and thus helps eliminate metabolic waste. It also decreases internal congestion.

Indications: Chronic joint and muscular rheumatism, gout, chronic neuralgia, sciatica

Contraindications: This wrap should not be used for heart patients, persons with diabetes or arteriosclerosis, or elderly persons.

Effects: Induces perspiration, detoxifies

Procedure: Prepare an ice bag, several hot water bottles, and linen sheet to steep in the hot water.

Prepare the table with a protective metallic blanket or sheet. On top place a large blanket. The blanket should overlap the edge of the table, and reach to the neck and over the feet like an envelope.

Fold a linen sheet in thirds, then lengthwise. Holding the ends, immerse it in an extremely hot water bath. Use rubber gloves to wring or squeeze out all of the water.

Place the wrung-out sheet over the dry blankets on the bed, and place the client on the table. Client should lie on his or her back with arms raised.

Apply a cold compress to the forehead and place an ice bag, wrapped in a dish towel, on heart.

Wrap the wet blanket over the right side of client's body. Bring arms down and quickly drape the left side of the wet blanket over the front of the body.

> **WARNING**
>
> The wrap increases the body temperature and pulse rate, so the pulse rate must be watched—especially with children and persons with vascular weakness. If pulse rate increases too rapidly, end the procedure.

Wrap the dry blankets(s) over the wet one, tucking it in at the shoulders and the feet. The metallic blanket sheet underneath the dry blankets will help retain the heat longer, and cause additional perspiration.

Place a series of hot water bottles at the feet, and along the sides of the body.

Client should drink large amounts of water and herb drinks.

Replace the forehead compress often so that it is always cold.

This pack can be applied for five to twenty minutes, depending on client's health. This wrap relaxes and soothes the muscles and helps to eliminate toxins.

Kneipp Body Wraps

Definition:

Every wrap has it own specific effect on the system. However, all wraps relax muscles, break up and absorb body toxins, and stimulate the whole organism. The major function of the wrap is to stimulate the skin, which in turn influences the body temperature, the nervous system, blood circulation, and the immune system. The effect of the wrap depends on its duration.

Procedure:

Heat Absorbing Cold Wrap

The cold wrap is used for reducing excess heat in the body (e.g., during infection or high fever). The wrap stays on until it is warm, usually twenty to thirty minutes. If the body temperature remains high, repeat the procedure.

Heat Retaining Cold Wrap

The cold wrap stays on until it has warmed up and has increased the circulation in the wrapped area without increasing perspiration. The wrap stays on for about an hour. The linen cloth must be wrung out thoroughly.

Perspiration Increasing Cold Wrap (Diaphoretic Wrap)

The wrap stays on until the client perspires profusely after one and a half to two hours. After perspiration begins, the wrap stays on for another fifteen minutes.

Types of Wrap:

Chest wrap, throat wrap, lumbar wrap, shawl wrap, foot wrap, short wrap, calf wrap, leg wrap, hand wrap, wet socks

Wrap Material:

Coarse linen cloth (interior cloth) lies on the skin, moist.

Cotton cloth (middle cloth) dry on the edges, two centimeters wider than the interior cloth.

Wool blanket (exterior cloth) dry on the edges, one centimeter smaller than the middle cloth.

Rules about Kneipp Body Wraps

1. They can be administered cold, tepid, or hot.

2. Additives such as vinegar, argillaceous earth (clay), salt, and dried herbs are effective.

3. Digestive tract should be cleared prior to wrap.

4. Hot wraps must be applied as hot as possible, while avoiding burns.

5. The wrap must be removed as quickly as possible.

6. After the wrap, the client should rest for thirty to sixty minutes.

7. The client should not read or watch television.

8. All wraps must fit snugly around the body.

9. Each cloth is wrapped in the same manner.

10. The room temperature where the wrap is applied should be 64°F.

11. Avoid drafts during the treatment.

12. Full body wraps should not be administered after meals.

Calf Wrap–Cold Temperature

Indications: Acute fever, local inflammation, venous inflammation, high blood pressure, overexertion after standing or walking for a long time, insomnia

Contraindications: Acute bladder or kidney infection, sciatica, onset of fever, cold feet

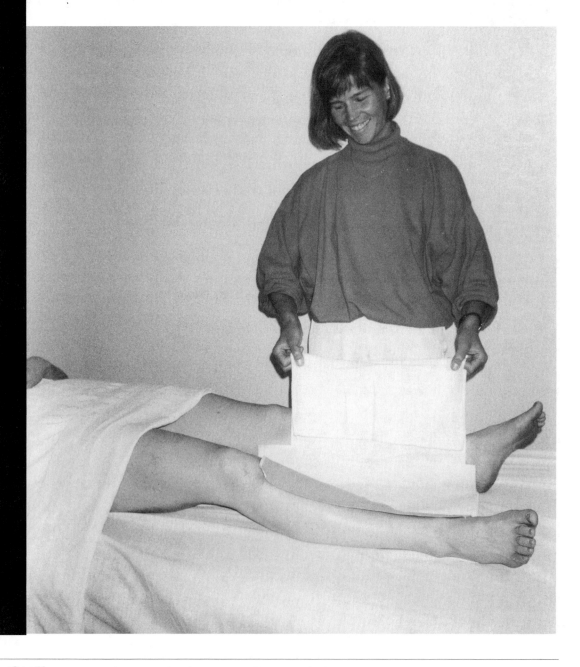

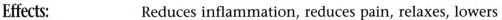

BODY WRAPS

Effects: Reduces inflammation, reduces pain, relaxes, lowers blood pressure

Equipment:

1 coarse linen cloth	12 in. × 30 in.
1 cotton cloth	13 in. × 30 in.
1 wool cloth	12.5 in. × 30 in.

Procedure: Dip coarse linen cloth wrap into cold water and then wring out.

Without wrinkling the cloth, wrap it snugly around the calf. The calf wrap covers the area from the ankle to the knee. Wrap the coarse linen (interior) tightly around the skin.

The next layer is the cotton cloth, which should be wrapped with a two-inch overlap.

The wool cloth is then wrapped as the exterior layer. Avoid extending the wool wrap over the cotton cloth.

After the treatment, bed rest is recommended.

Duration: Approximately fifteen to twenty minutes, or as soon as the wrap feels warm to the client

Wet Socks

Indications: Insomnia, varicose veins

Contraindications: Menstruation, acute bladder or kidney infection, cold feet, oversensitivity to cold

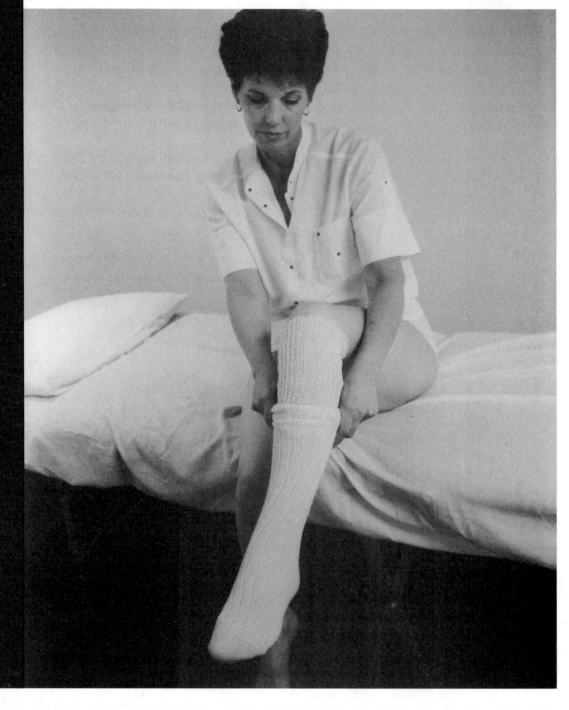

Equipment:	Linen socks, wool socks
Procedure:	Dip coarse linen socks into cold water, then wring them out.
	Put on wet linen socks, and then put on wool socks.
Duration:	To enhance sleep: fifteen to twenty minutes or as soon as the socks feel warm to the client (can be worn all night).
	For varicose veins or circulation problems in the legs: the socks should be removed before they become warm.
Herbal Additives:	Meadow flower essential oil

Chest Wrap–Cold Temperature

Indications: Acute bronchitis, inflammation of the lungs (pneumonia), pleurisy

Contraindications: Oversensitivity to cold

Effects: Reduces inflammation, a short cooling off period causes a re-warming of the body and increases the blood circulation, breaks down bronchial secretion, reduces fever and pain

Equipment:
1 coarse linen cloth	16 × 75 in.
1 cotton cloth	19 × 75 in.
1 wool cloth	17 × 75 in.

Procedure: Dip the coarse linen cloth into cold water and then wring out.

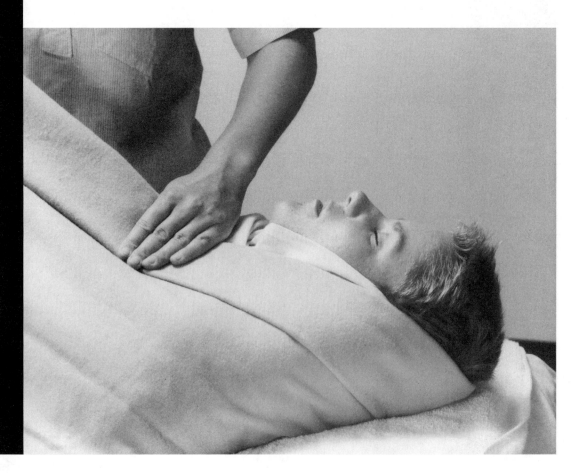

BODY WRAPS

The cold moist chest wrap reaches from the armpit to the pelvic crest. The wrap must fit snugly. Wrap the coarse linen cloth tightly around the skin.

The next layer is the cotton cloth, which should be wrapped leaving a $1^1/_2$-inch overlap. The final layer is the wool cloth, which should not touch the skin.

After wrapping, rest is recommended.

Duration: Forty-five to seventy-five minutes, or as soon as the wrap feels warm to the client

> ### NOTE
> Chest wrap enhances the effect of oral cold medication. The goal of the treatment is to create heat. Herbal additives and clay water can be used.

BODY WRAPS

Chest Wrap–Hot Temperature

Indications: Chronic bronchitis

Contraindications: Fever

Effects: Bronchodilation, enhances bronchial secretion

Equipment:
1 coarse linen cloth	16 × 75 in.
1 cotton cloth	19 × 75 in.
1 wool cloth	17 × 75 in.

Procedure: Dip the coarse linen cloth into very hot water, and then wring out.

The hot moist chest wrap covers the area from the armpit to the pelvic crest. The wrap must fit snugly.

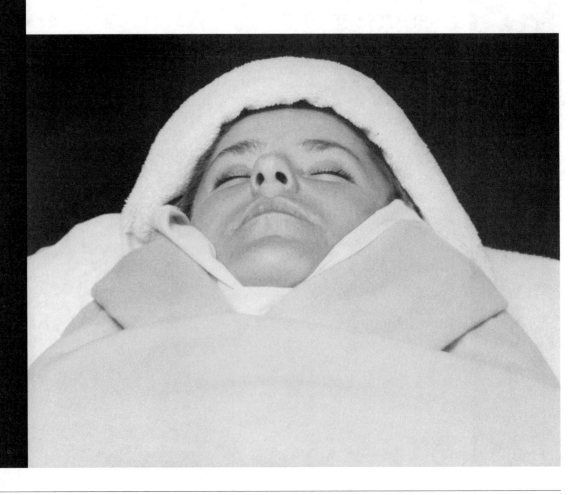

Wrap the coarse linen cloth tightly around the skin.

The next layer is the cotton cloth, which should be wrapped leaving a $1^{1}/_{2}$-inch overlap.

The final layer is the wool cloth, which should not touch the skin.

After wrapping, bed rest is recommended.

Duration: The wrap stays on as long as it feels warm to the client

> ### NOTE
>
> It is optional to rub the chest and back with an essential oil prior to the wrap. Herbal additives can be used in hot water.

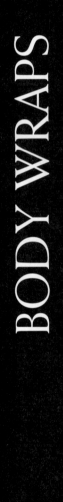
Throat Wrap–
Cold Temperature

Indications: Acute throat inflammation

Contraindications: Onset of a cold or a fever

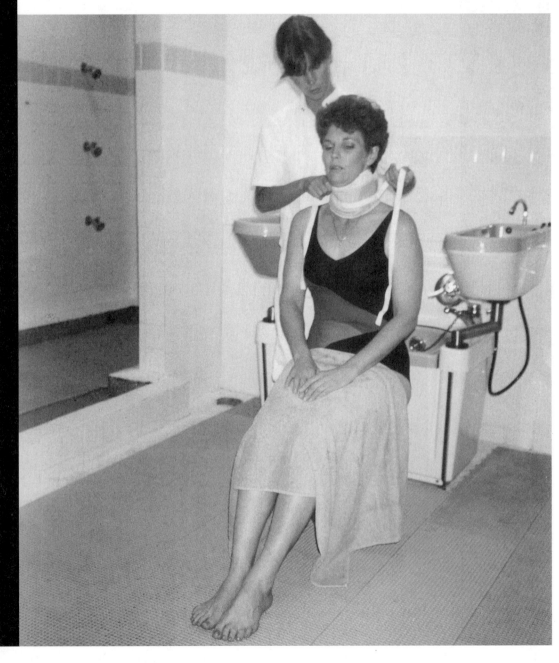

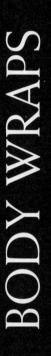

BODY WRAPS

Effects:	Withdrawing heat
Equipment:	1 coarse linen cloth 4 × 28 in.
	1 cotton cloth 6 × 28 in.
	1 wool cloth 5 × 28 in.

Procedure:

Dip coarse linen cloth into cold water and squeeze it out.

Wrap the coarse linen cloth tightly around the skin. The cold wrap should cover the neck completely.

The next layer is the cotton cloth, which should be wrapped leaving a $1^1/_2$-inch overlap.

The final layer is the wool cloth, which should not touch the skin.

After wrapping, bed rest is recommended.

Duration:

Acute processes: When the wrap no longer feels cold to the client, remove the wrap and apply a second wrap immediately. The wrap can be applied twice a day (once in the morning and once in the evening).

WARNING

If pain increases during the treatment, remove the wrap immediately.

Lumbar Wrap–
Cold Temperature

Indications: Chronic indigestion, abdominal and mucous membrane inflammation, high blood pressure, insomnia

Contraindications: Menstruation, acute kidney infection

Effects: Stabilizes digestive organs, enhances sleep, relaxes autonomic nervous system, reduces pain

Equipment:

1 coarse linen cloth	16 × 75 in.
1 cotton cloth	20 × 75 in.
1 wool cloth	18 × 75 in.

Procedure: Dip the coarse linen cloth into cold water and then wring out.

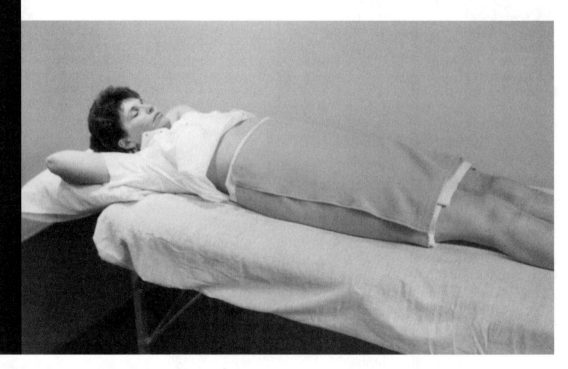

> **NOTE**
>
> If the client does not warm up after about ten minutes, offer a cup of hot tea or a hot water bottle.

The wrap covers the lower trunk and upper part of the thighs. The wrap must fit snugly. Wrap the coarse linen cloth tightly around the skin.

The next layer is the cotton cloth, which should be wrapped with a 1½-inch overlap.

The exterior layer is the wool cloth, which should not touch the skin.

After wrapping, bed rest is recommended.

Duration: Forty-five to seventy-five minutes

CHAPTER 13

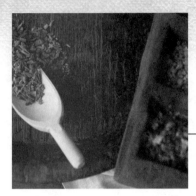

BODY PACKS

Mustard Pack

Definition: Mustard powder, when made into a paste with a touch of water and flour and applied in a cloth onto lightly oiled skin, has the unique power of bringing blood to the surface of the skin. It quickly heats up the area, and, as the blood rushes to the skin surface, even the worst congestion diminishes.

Indications: Internal congestion, lumbago pain, neuritis, poor local circulation, bronchitis, sciatica

Procedure: Prepare a large linen or cotton cloth by folding the cloth in thirds.

In a bowl, mix one cup of dry, powdered mustard with tepid water until it has a creamy consistency. Increase the amount of powder according to the amount of poultice needed.

Place the mustard paste on a paper towel. Fold the towel and make a pack, and place it in the folded linen or cotton cloth. Heat the pack by placing a hot water bottle on it.

If the client has sensitive skin, oil the skin lightly with olive or vegetable oil.

Place a thin cloth on the area, and apply the mustard pack.

Cover the area with a blanket.

At first the heat may seem intense, but then it lessens. As the skin becomes very red, the pack can be transferred from area to area, from the front of the chest to the upper back (in case of bronchitis) or to other areas of intense pain.

Duration: Apply the pack to each area for two to ten minutes. The entire treatment should last a half-hour.

Hot and Cold Fango (Mud) and Clay Packs

Definition: Hot sand, hot fango packs, and clay packs have been used for centuries by different cultures to relieve joint pain. The material used is either organic volcanic ash, peat from bogs, mineral sea mud, or clay from high mineral areas. All of these substances are available in powder form. Fango (mud) packs have extracting ability because the mineral content increases the heat and chemical action on the skin. Because clay and/or earth draw out poisons, such packs not only soften the skin and release tension around joints, but also absorb internal toxic or pathogenic material.

Indications: Chronic rheumatism, chronic neuralgia, chronic pain, non-acute arthritis, muscle spasms, chronic sciatica

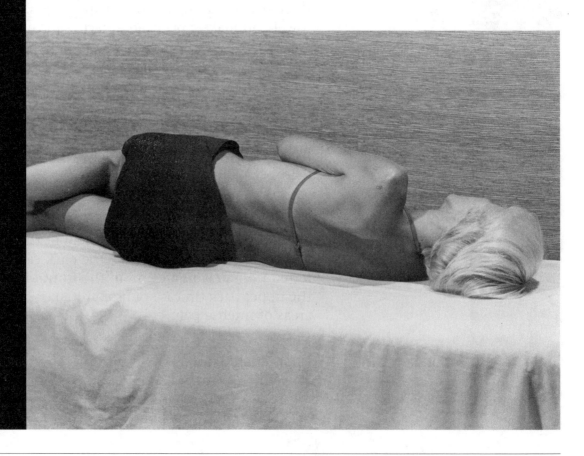

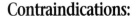BODY PACKS

Contraindications: Small applications of clay or mud will vitalize the entire body, but immersion mineral mud baths are contraindicated in cases of heart disease, diabetes, high blood pressure, or arteriosclerosis.

Procedure: Heat up the mud powder. Add water to soften it. Spread this in a one- or two-inch thickness on a soft cotton cloth, slightly larger than the area you wish to cover.

Place the hot mud directly on the hurt area.

Cover the area with a dry lightweight cloth. Leave on until it dries (fifteen to thirty minutes).

Rinse off with warm water, then splash with a little cool water.

Remove the dried mud by sponging or showering it off.

Follow with a rain or needle shower.

Dry gently with a mild cloth.

If the body is still heated, keep the area warm and dry afterward.

Fango Moor Pack Ascend

BODY PACKS

Ingredients: Natural Moor-Peloid from the moorfields of northern Germany

Indications for Hot Pack Application: Subacute and chronic conditions of rheumatism, degenerative joint and spinal conditions, soft tissue rheumatism, postacute traumas of joints and muscles, lack of functional blood circulation, chronic pain, discomfort in the abdominal region

Contraindications for Hot Pack Application: Acute inflammation, trauma, bleeding, edema, insufficiencies in vascular capillaries and vessels, elevated body temperature, fever, sensitive skin areas, acute skin conditions, skin burns

Indications for Cold Pack Application: Acute conditions of rheumatism, degenerative joint and spinal conditions, soft tissue rheumatism, acute traumas of joints and muscles, acute inflammation of organs in the abdominal region, augmentive therapy in venous and lymphatic vascular symptoms, fever

Contraindications for Cold Pack Application: Insufficiencies in vascular capillaries and vessels, local and general skin sensitivity to cold

Procedure: Apply pack with fleece side to the skin.

Hot pack application temperature is 107°F or more, according to tolerance.

Cold pack application temperature is 60°F or less, according to tolerance.

Apply pack for twenty to thirty minutes.

Client should rest after application for twenty to thirty minutes.

Parafango (Paraffin Fango) Pack

Definition: Investigations aimed at improving the thermo-physical conditions of fango, which would make the application easier and raise the basic hygienic conditions when thermal fango packs were applied, led to the development of Parafango by Professor Hesse in Hamburg, Germany. Introduced as a treatment in 1952, the preparation has since become widely known in practice and literature in Europe.

Parafango is compounded of dried fango and paraffins with different fusing points. It also contains minute additions of talcum and magnesium oxide in order to prevent the fango from precipitating in the melted paraffins, as well as to heighten the plasticity and the malleability of the material. Parafango melts at (140°F–158°F) to an easy-to-spread paste that, exactly within the range of its temperature of application, constitutes an extremely plastic mass that is easily molded to any part of the body at 122°F. The application of hot Parafango packs on parts of the body's surface is a purely thermal process.

Indications: Inflammatory rheumatism (declining acute rheumatism and rheumatoid arthritis, anchylosis spondylitis or M. Bechterew), degenerative rheumatism (osteo-

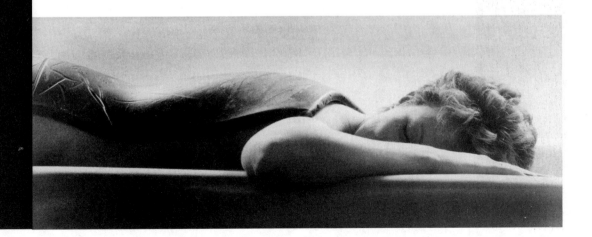

arthritis, intervertebral discopathies, non-articular rheumatism such as fibrositis myalgia, painful shoulder), dermatology (psoriatic arthropathy, scleroderma)

Contraindications: Acute neuritis, acute primary rheumatoid arthritis, recent thrombophlebitis and eczema, all forms of heart and circulation deficiencies, high grade hypertension, angina pectoris, distinct vegetative dystonia, and convalescence

Procedure: **Local packings:** On one or two larger joints, a small area of torso.

Part packs: On three or four large joints, entire extremities, back and abdomen, or pelvic packs.

Large packs: Entire extremities, back with abdominal pack.

BODY PACKS

Alpine Flower Haypack

Indications: Area with muscular tension and/or joint discomfort, degeneration of the joints, degeneration of the spine, or acute bronchitis

Contraindications: Heart disease, inflamed treatment area

Effects: Relaxes, increases blood circulation, reduces pain, calms

Equipment:
1 wool blanket
1 linen cloth
1 meadow flower herbal pack

Procedure: Moisten the herbal pack with water.

Place herbal pack in a steamer or in a hydroinfuser. Steam the pack for approximately thirty minutes.

Remove the haypack carefully from the steamer and shake it with both hands.

Apply the haypack carefully.

Observe the skin's reaction to the pack.

Gradually wrap tighter.

After wrapping, cover client with a blanket.

Remove the pack before it cools down (usually forty-five minutes).

Have client rest for thirty to sixty minutes after the treatment.

> **NOTE**
>
> Be careful not to burn the skin, especially when haypack has just been removed from the steamer.

Neck Haypack– Hot Temperature

BODY PACKS

Indications:	Tightness in the neck, cervical syndrome
Contraindications:	Neuritis, inflammation of the skin in the treatment area
Effects:	Relaxes muscles, reduces spasms, increases blood circulation, stimulates metabolism, reduces pain
Equipment:	1 wool blanket 1 linen cloth 1 meadow flower haypack
Procedure:	Apply the hot haypack tightly onto the neck. Be careful not to burn the skin. In order to prevent heat from escaping, wrap the haypack snugly. Leave on as long as the pack feels warm.

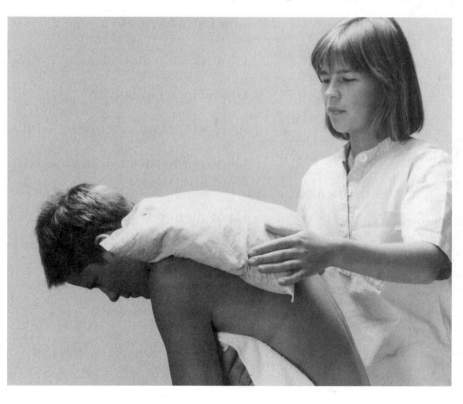

Lumbar Haypack– Hot Temperature

Indications:	Chronic coxarthrosis, chronic lumbago
Contraindications:	Acute lumbago, inflammation in the area of treatment
Effects:	Relaxes muscles, reduces spasms, stimulates blood circulation, calms, reduces pain
Equipment:	1 wool blanket 1 linen cloth 1–2 meadow flower haypacks

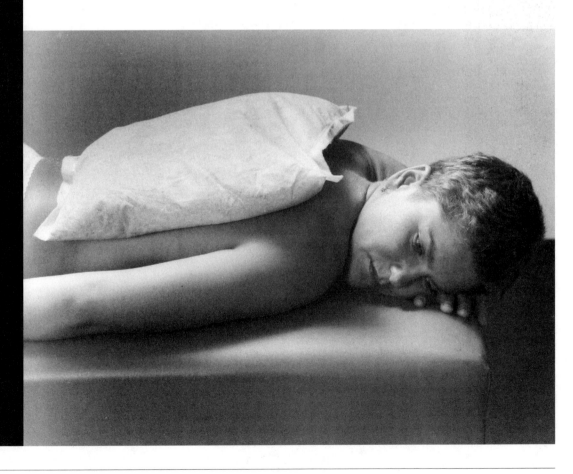

Procedure:

Apply the haypack carefully on the client.

Fasten haypack tightly and be careful not to burn the skin.

In order to prevent heat from escaping, wrap the haypack snugly.

The client can lie sideways or lie comfortably on the back.

Leave on as long as the haypack feels warm to the client.

BODY PACKS

CHAPTER 14

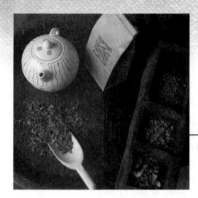

HOT COMPRESSES

General Description

HOT COMPRESSES

Indications:	Muscular tension in cervical, lumbar, and abdominal areas
Contraindications:	Inflammation in the treatment area
Effects:	Relaxes muscles, reduces spasms, increases blood circulation, stimulates metabolism, reduces pain, calms
Equipment:	1 coarse linen cloth 1 cotton cloth 1 wool cloth 2 towels
Procedure:	Fold the coarse linen sheet and dip into hot water. Remove the folded sheet carefully from the hot water. Roll in a dry towel. Wring excess water out of towel. Fold wet compress in a dry towel. Apply hot compress to the respective body part (e.g., neck, stomach, lower back). In order to prevent heat from escaping, wrap client snugly. Leave compress on until hot compress cools down. Client should rest for sixty to seventy-five minutes after the treatment.

> **WARNING**
>
> Be careful not to burn the skin.

Abdominal Compress— Hot Temperature

HOT COMPRESSES

Indications: Bloating, spasms in the treatment area

Contraindications: Inflammation in the abdominal area, pregnancy

Effects: Relaxes muscles, increases blood circulation

Equipment: 1 coarse linen cloth
1 cotton cloth
1 wool cloth
2 towels

Procedure: Dip the folded, coarse linen sheet into hot water. Remove the folded sheet carefully from the water and roll in a dry towel.

Wring out excess water.

Fold wet compress in a dry towel.

Apply hot pack to the respective body part.

In order to prevent heat from escaping, wrap client snugly.

Leave compress on as long as it feels warm.

The client should rest for at least one hour after treatment.

> **WARNING**
>
> Be careful not to burn the skin.

Abdominal Compress— Cold Temperature

Indications:	Constipation, indigestion, fevers
Contraindications:	Menstruation, pregnancy
Effects:	Promotes digestion, reduces inflammation
Equipment:	1 coarse linen cloth 1 linen cloth 1 wool cloth
Procedure:	Dip the folded, coarse linen sheet into cold water. Remove the folded sheet and wring out excess water. Apply the cold pack to the respective body part. Wrap the client. The client should rest for at least one hour after the treatment.

The Hot Roll

A hot rolled towel is a practical means of applying heat to a small area of the body. This is a popular treatment for athletic injuries because the necessary materials are readily available.

Five medium-sized towels are necessary. Fold four of the towels lengthwise (place the fifth towel aside, it will be used later). The first towel is rolled up like an elastic bandage (a spiral-shaped point should protrude along one edge and a funnel-shaped hollow is formed on the other side). The second towel is wrapped cylindrically around the first, but with the edges even with the final turns of the first towel. The point and the funnel are not enlarged. The third and fourth towels are then wrapped around the first two towels. The towels should be wrapped as tightly as possible so that water is unable to drip out. After all four towels have been wrapped, pour a liter of boiling water into the funnel-shaped form.

The four towels completely absorb the water. Now the fifth towel is wrapped around the roll, so that a bit of the towel extends on all sides. This is important, so that the therapist can get a good grasp on the towel. Their use is then relatively simple. The pack is placed against the area to be treated using gentle pressure. After a brief period of contact, it is removed for a moment and then replaced. The process continues in this rhythmic form until the body has become accustomed to the heat. After this point has been reached, the towel roll is left on the body for longer periods of time, and finally is no longer removed. Gentle massaging movements are included in the treatment. There is no chance of cooling, first because the skin maintains a high temperature and second, because the towel roll is repeatedly run over the entire skin surface even though smaller areas are treated at short intervals throughout the treatment. After even a short time, the skin becomes deeply flushed, and remains so for quite some time. When the outer towel is no longer hot enough, it is slowly unwrapped.

The hot rolled towel maintains its temperature practically unchanged in its interior throughout. Gradually the towels are unrolled. The rate at which the towels are unwrapped depends on how fast the outer layer cools and on the sensitivity of the individual client. The therapist spreads the last towel over the treated area and leaves it there until the client no longer feels its warmth. Treatment with hot rolled towels lasts about fifteen minutes. Among the advantages of this form of treatment is that it permits individual variations. It also permits treatment in a wide range of temperatures.

The hot rolled towel is an excellent treatment for athletes with over-strained spinal columns.

Treatment with incandescent irradiation and hot moist towels is similar to the treatment of hot rolled towels. Athletes prefer this treatment because it is simple to administer. The warm, moist towel is laid on the treated body part. Then the incandescent lamp is placed over it. The length of application is fifteen to twenty minutes.

HOT COMPRESSES

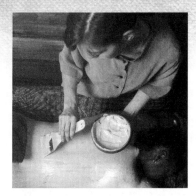

CHAPTER 15

HERBAL AND MINERAL BODY MASK AND WRAP THERAPIES

Volcanic Fango Body Mask

Definition: This is a mineral-rich body mask utilizing the revitalizing effects of fango.

Procedure: Place blanket, electric blanket, plastic sheet, and linen sheet on treatment table. Turn electric blanket to medium setting. Have knee bolster, a head pillow covered with a towel, ice water, glasses, and drinking straws available.

A short stay in the sauna to elevate body temperature and to relax client is optional.

Prepare the Dead Sea fango mask at this time. To prepare the fango mask, pour six ounces of fango mask into a bowl. Heat to about 102°F (about one minute in a microwave oven or longer in a hydrocollator or bowl of hot water).

Have the client lie down on his or her stomach and apply mask, beginning with the legs. Cover the whole body.

Move fast so the client does not get cold.

Have client turn over and cover the front of the client's body with the rest of the mask. Wrap client tightly in plastic sheet, then wrap with electric blanket and blanket.

After fifteen minutes, unwrap client and have client take a shower.

Valerian Herbal Wrap

MASKS AND WRAPS

Definition: This popular European treatment relaxes the skin and body and leaves the client refreshed.

Procedure: Place blanket and/or electric blanket and linen sheet on treatment tables. Turn electric blanket to low setting. Have knee bolster, a head pillow covered with a towel, ice water, glasses, and drinking straws available.

Prepare valerian herbal wrap application. Note that only a small amount (one ounce) is needed for the whole body.

Have the client lie down on his or her stomach and apply the valerian herbal wrap gel, beginning with the legs.

Cover the whole body.

Move fast so the client does not get cold.

Have client turn over and cover the front of the client's body.

Wrap client in linen sheet, then wrap with electric blanket and/or blanket.

Play soft relaxing music. Let client relax.

A scalp and/or foot massage is an optional addition to this treatment.

After twenty minutes, unwrap client and mist the client with rosewater.

> **NOTE**
>
> This is a no-shower treatment.

Seaweed Body Wrap

Definition: This is a light green blend of micronized laminaria digitata and lithothamnium calcarium powders from the coastal waters of the Brittany province of France.

Ingredients: 100% pure seaweed powders

Indications: Used as a paste to perform body wraps and masks to treat cellulite and other figure complaints

Contraindications: No known contraindications. However, avoid inhaling powder during mixing.

Effects: Features the minerals magnesium, potassium, and calcium to restore cellular balance and fight the symptoms of bloat. The trace elements silica, zinc, selenium, and iodine nourish skin, scavenge free radicals, and increase metabolism. Algini acid is an elasticizing agent and emollient, while beta-carotene provides vitamin A for skin vitality. A balanced concentrate of the ocean's nutrients, this nourishes skin, tones and detoxifies tissues, and reduces bloat.

Procedure: Place a metallic blanket, electric blanket, and plastic sheet on table.

Thirty minutes before treatment, turn on electric blanket. Have knee bolster, a head pillow covered with a towel, ice water, glasses, and drinking straws available.

Have client take a warm shower.

After the shower, recommend a short stay in the sauna to elevate body temperature and to relax client.

Mix seaweed powder into a paste.

Have client stand next to treatment table without

clothes or, if uncomfortable, with a swimsuit, and proceed to dry-brushing (always stroke upwards towards the heart) with a loofah sponge to slough off dead skin cells and to stimulate blood to the surface.

After dry-brushing, have client lie down on stomach and massage seaweed body mask cream onto legs and buttocks (or where cellulite occurs).

Cover the whole body with seaweed mask.

Have client turn over and cover the front of the client's body with the rest of the seaweed mask.

Wrap client tightly in a plastic sheet.

Then wrap with electric blanket and metallic blanket.

Turn off lights. Play soft relaxing music.

Place an ice-cold damp towel on the client's forehead and offer a glass of cold water.

Let client relax.

Check client every ten minutes.

After thirty to forty minutes, unwrap client and have client take a shower (preferably cold).

CHAPTER 16

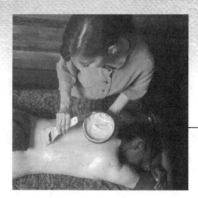

EXFOLIATION TREATMENTS

Salt Glow

EXFOLIATION TREATMENTS

Definition: A salt glow provides increased vasodilatation without heating or cooling the body, stimulates circulation, increases nerve activity, and increases the sense of well-being and feeling of vitality. It also removes dead skin.

Indications: To be used on clients who do not react well to heat or cold; sluggish circulation, frequent colds, low blood pressure, general weakness, low endurance

Contraindications: Skin lesions or sores, eczema

Equipment: Use two to four pounds (one to two kilograms) fine kiln salt, sheet, towels, shower

Procedure: Add just enough water to the salt to make it sticky (not too dry or too wet).

Pre-wet the skin that is to be treated.

Rub the skin briskly with salt until the skin is pink.

Do all parts of the body in turn: arms and hands, shoulders, chest and abdomen, back, thighs and legs, and feet.

Remove the salt using a shower, bath, or affusion using water of a cool but pleasant temperature.

Dry client well and keep body warm.

Body Scrub

Definition: This is a gentle exfoliating process using honey and almond scrub and a loofah sponge. This treatment cleans the skin, removes cellular debris, and, through the moisturizing properties of honey, leaves the skin invigorated.

Procedure: A short stay in the sauna or a warm shower before the scrub is optional.

Have client lie face down on stomach and wet down body.

Apply scrub with hands, beginning with legs. Cover the whole body.

Use loofah to scrub body in gentle circular motion.

Rinse and have client turn over.

Repeat procedure.

Pat dry.

Misting the body with a skin toner is optional.

CHAPTER 17

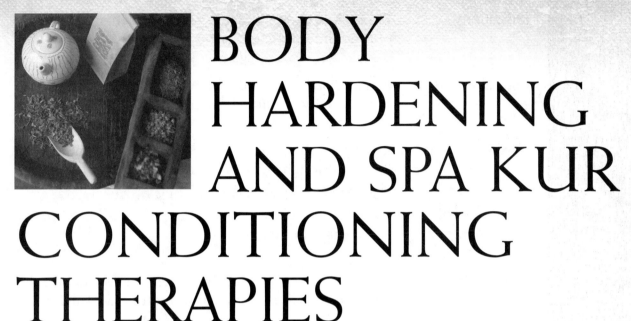

BODY HARDENING AND SPA KUR CONDITIONING THERAPIES

Dry-Brushing

Indications: Hypertension, low blood pressure, toughening effects of the skin, mild varicose veins, insomnia

Contraindications: Acne, inflammatory skin ailments, skin injuries, hyperactivity, inflamed varicose veins

Effects: Regenerates and tones skin. Stimulates skin metabolism and sloughing, stimulates circulation with reflex effects on internal organs

Equipment: Brush (natural bristles)

Procedure: Brush the lower body in this order: right foot and sole; right calf (brush in a circular fashion); right thigh (first exterior then interior).

Repeat procedure on left leg.

Brush buttocks.

Turn to the upper body: right hand and arm (exterior then interior, lengthwise).

Repeat procedure on left arm.

Brush the chest towards sternum.

Brush abdomen clockwise.

Brush neck towards shoulder.

Then brush the upper back, lower back, and face (use soft bristle brush).

Brush until skin appears red, usually five minutes.

After the dry-brushing, cold washing, snow-rubbing, oiling the skin, or exercises are recommended.

> **NOTE**
>
> Best performed in the morning after getting up. Evening usage can cause sleep disturbances.

Airbath

Indications: General body defense insufficiency, psoriasis vulgaris, poor healing, infected skin

Contraindications: Acute eczema, tuberculosis, sun allergies, hepatitis, hyperthyroidism. Client cannot receive treatment if under medication that causes photosensitivity, autonomic hyperactivity, underpigmentation, cardiac inflammation, acute arthritic inflammatory diseases, and mucous membrane inflammations

Effects: Improves general immunity, stimulates metabolism

Equipment: Plenty of fluid intake, sunscreen

Procedure: Natural shade: Trees, bushes. Cover body parts alternately.

To cool down: cool bath, shower, washing, or affusion. Pauses slow cooling as indicated above.

Special Considerations:

1. Never jump into cold water without previously cooling down because of possible cardiac arrest.

2. Be careful in high altitudes or when near water (increased strength of rays).

3. Differentiate between natural sunlight and artificial rays.

NOTE

If client has a fever or heat stroke, pay close attention during the cooling phase and washings, and monitor liquid intake. If client has a sunstroke, gentle cooling and a physician's assistance are recommended. Prevent injury with a sensible, well-dosed application.

Dew Walking

Indications:	Mild arterial circulation disorders (first degree), venous disturbances of the legs, morning fatigue
Contraindications:	Menstruation, urinary infections, bladder and kidney ailments, sciatic pains, shivers, cold feet, arterial occlusion disorders (second to fourth degree)
Effects:	Promotes circulation, strengthens foot and calf muscles, strengthens veins, stabilizes autonomic system, prevents infection
Equipment:	Dew-moistened lawn
Procedure:	Walk on dew-moistened grass for about five minutes with warm feet. Stop if a cutting pain occurs.
Duration:	Approximately ten minutes
Special Considerations:	Avoid undercooling.

BODY HARDENING

Water Treading

BODY HARDENING

Indications:	Insomnia, mild arterial circulation disorders (first degree), venous disturbances in the legs, venous circulation disorders, conditions resulting from thrombophlebitis, disturbances with warmth regulation, susceptibility to infections, tendency to hypertension, cardiac neurosis, cardiac stenosis, headaches stemming from the blood vessels, dazed states, climactic sensitivity
Contraindications:	Menstruation, urinary infections, bladder and kidney ailments, female pelvic disorders, arterial circulation disorders (second to fourth degree), chills, cold legs and feet
Effects:	Strengthens the veins, influences venous return followed by warming, stimulates circulation (hyperemia), induces sleep, soothes, stimulates metabolism
Equipment:	Treading basin, bathtub, river, etc. (the water level should be at least one hand width below the knee).
Procedure:	With bare legs, "stork walk" by lifting leg out of water with each step.
	Can also be done seated.
	Stop if cutting pain occurs.
	Wipe water off and put socks and shoes on immediately.
	Reheat body by walking.
Duration:	Depends on water temperature; approximately thirty to sixty seconds.
Special Considerations:	Avoid undercooling. Reheating is necessary (wearing warm socks to bed or exercising).

Snow Walking

Indications: Chronic headaches, susceptibility to infection, fatigue

Contraindications: Chills, cold feet, menstruation, female abdominal disorders, urinary infections, arterial circulation disorders (second to fourth degree)

Effects: Stimulates circulation, refreshes

Equipment: Soft snow, wool socks

Procedure: Begin by walking in the snow for a few seconds or until cutting sensation occurs.

After training you will be able to walk in the snow for about three minutes.

The walk should be followed by reheating (e.g., wearing wool socks, brisk walking, rubbing).

Duration: Approximately three minutes

Special Considerations: Perform in soft snow only (hazard of cuts if performed on hard snow). Avoid slipping by walking carefully. Do not come in contact with metal or remain standing in the snow (may get frostbitten).

SAMPLE KNEIPP SPA KUR THERAPY PROGRAM

	EARLY MORNING	LATE MORNING	AFTERNOON
WEEK 1			
Monday	Upper Body Washing	Arm Affusion, Alternate, and Face, Cold	Knee Affusion, Cold
Tuesday	Lower Body Washing	Chest Affusion, Alternate, and Face, Cold, Alternate	Knee Affusion
Wednesday	Whole Body Washing	³/₄ Bath Hay Flowers after Full Body Affusion, Cold	
Thursday	Haypack, Neck	Alternate Leg Affusion	Arm Affusion, Alternate
Friday	Whole Body Washing	Chest Affusion, Alternate, and Face	Footbath, Alternate
Saturday	Haypack, Lumbar	Lumbar Affusion, Increasing Temperature	
WEEK 2			
Monday	Whole Body Washing	³/₄ Herbal Bath, after Full Body Affusion, Cold	Knee Affusion, Cold
Tuesday	Haypack, Neck	Neck Affusion, Increasing Temperature	Knee Affusion, Cold
Wednesday		Arm Bath, Increasing Temperature	
Thursday	Calf Wrap Cold	Chest Affusion, Alternate Temperature	Knee Affusion, Cold
Friday	Haypack, Neck	Neck Affusion, Increasing Temperature	Knee Affusion, Cold
Saturday	Whole Body Washing	³/₄ Herbal Bath, after Full Body Affusion, Cold	
WEEK 3			
Monday	Upper Body Washing	Knee Affusion, Alternate Temperature	Arm Bath, Cold
Tuesday	Lower Body Washing	Arm Affusion, Cold, and Face	Knee Affusion, Alternate Temperature
Wednesday		³/₄ Herbal Bath, after Full Body Affusion, Cold	
Thursday	Upper Body Washing	Foot Bath, Alternate Temperature	
Friday	Haypack, Neck		Knee Affusion, Cold
Saturday		Arm and Face Affusion, Alternate Temperature	

REFERENCES

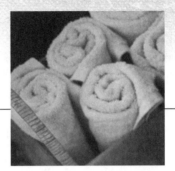

Abrahams, V. C., S. M. Hilton, and A. Zbrozyna. Active muscle dilation produced by stimulation of the brain stem: Its significance in the defense reaction. J. Physiol. (Lond.) 154, 491–513 (1960).

Abramson, D. I. Indirect vasodilatation in thermotherapy. Arch. Phys. Med. Rehabil. 46, 412–415 (1965).

Adolph, E. F. General and specific characteristic of physiological adaptations. Am. J. Physiol. 184, 18–28 (1956).

Alberti, B., M. Schlepper, K. Westermann, and E. Witzleb. Ober den Tonus unter dem EinfluB von thermisehen Reizen. Z. Angew. Bader und Klimaheilkd 13, 453–471 (1966).

Aschoff, J. Pfluegers Arch. 248, 171 (1944) Zit, nach Bildebrandt, G. Zur Physiologie der Muskeldurchblutung des Menschen. Arch. Phys. Ther. 10, 217–223 (1958).

Barcroft, J., and W. King. The effect of temperature on the dissociation curve of blood. J. Physiol. 39, 374–384 (1909).

Bayliss, W. M. On the local reactions of the arterial wall to changes in internal pressure. J. Physiol. (Lond.) 28, 220–231 (1904).

Benson, T. B., and E. P. Copp. The effects of therapeutic forms of heat and ice on the pain threshold of the normal shoulder. Rheumatol. Rehabil. 13, 101–104 (1974).

Bergmann, K. G. Ch. L.: Arch. Anat. Physiol. 300 (1845) zit. Nach Aschoff, J., Wechselwirkungen zwischen Kern und Schale in Warmehaushalt. Arch. Physikal. Ther. 8, 113–133 (1956).

Betz, E. Ober die Vasomotorik bei Ischiaserkrankungen. Arch. Physikal. Ther. 6, 29–37 (1954).

Bohannon, R. W. Whirlpool versus whirlpool rinse for removal of bacteria from a venous stasis ulcer. Phys. Ther. 62(3), 304–308 (1982).

Botell, P. M., R. Parker, E. J. Henley, et al. Comparison of in vivo temperatures produced by hydrotherapy paraffin wax treatment and fluidotherapy. Phys. Ther. 60, 1273–1276 (1980).

Brendstrip, P., K. Jespersen, and G. Asboe-Hansen. Morphological and chemical connective tissue changes in fibrositic muscles. Annals of Rheumatology 16, 438 (1957).

Bruggemann, W. Die Kneipptherapie in der Pravention von gefaBkrankheiten. Pharm. Unserer Zeit 4, 109–116 (1972).

—Die Kneipptherapie. Z. Physikal. Med. 5, 1–12 (1976).

Bungaj, R. The cooling, analgesic, and re-warming effects of ice massage on localized skin. Phys. Ther. 55(1), 11–19 (1975).

Clarke, R. S. J., R. F. Hellon, and A. R. Lind. Vascular reactions in the human forearm to cold. Clin. Sci. 17, 165–179 (1958).

Coles, D. R., and G. C. Patterson. Capacity and distensibility of blood vessels of human hand. J. Physiol. (Lond.) 135, 163–170 (1957).

Cooper, K. E., McK, Kerslake D. Abolition of nervous reflex vasodilatation of sympathectomy of the heated area. J. Physiol. (Lond.) 119, 18029 (1953).

Crockford, G. W., R. F. Hellon, and J. Parkhouse. Thermal vasomotor response in human skin mediated by local mechanisms. J. Physiol. 161, 10–15 (1962).

Folkow, B., B. Johansson, and B. Oberge. A hypothalamic structure with a marked inhibitory effect on tonic sympathetic activity. Acta Physiol. Scand. 47, 262–270 (1959).

Folkow, B., S. Melander, and B. Oberg. The range of effect of the sympathetic vasodilator fibres with regard to the consecutive sections of the muscle vessels. Acta Physiol. Scand. 53, 7–22 (1961).

Fox, H. H., and S. M. Hilton. Bradykinin formation in human skin as a factor in heat vasodilatation. J. Physiol. 142, 219 (1958).

Fox. R., and H. Wyatt. Cold induced vasodilatation in various areas of the body surface in man. J. Physiol. 162(1), 289-297 (1962).

Guyton, A. C. Textbook of Medical Physiology, eighth ed. Philadelphia: WB Saunders, 1991.

Keating, W. R. Effect of low temperatures on the responses of arteries to constrictor drugs. J. Physiol. (Lond.) 142, 395–405 (1958).

—The effect of general chilling on the vasodilatation response to cold. J. Physiol. 139(3), 497–507 (1957).

—Survival in Cold Water. Oxford: Blackwell, 1978.

Kerslake, D. McK., and K. E. Cooper. Vasodilatation in the hand in response to heating the skin elsewhere. Clin. Sci. 9, 31–47 (1950).

Kidd, B. S. L., and S. M. Lyon. Distensibility of blood vessels of the human calf determined by graded venous congestion. J. Physiol. (Lond.) 140, 122–128 (1958).

Klingelhofer, R. Langsschnittuntersuchungen der akustischen und optischen Reaktionszeitan zur Beurteilung der aktivierenden Kurbchandlung. Med. Inaug. Diss. Marburg/Lahn, 1973.

Lee, J. M., M. P. Warren, and S. M. Mason. Effects of ice on nerve conduction velocity. Physiotherapy 64, 2–6 (1978).

Lehmann, J. F., G. Brunner, and R. Stow. Pain threshold measurements after therapeutic application of ultrasound, microwaves and infrared. Arch. Phys. Med. Rehabil. 39, 560–565 (1958).

Lehmann, J. F., and B. J. DeLateur. Therapeutic heat. In Lehmann, J. F. (ed), Therapeutic Heat and Cold, fourth ed. Baltimore: Williams & Wilkins, 1990.

Lewis, T. Observations upon the reactions of the vessels of the human skin to cold. Heart 15, 177–208 (1930).

Magnes, J., T. Garret, and D. Erickson. Swelling of the upper extremity during whirlpool baths. Arch. Phys. Med. Rehabl. 51, 297–299 (1970).

Mayer, D. J., and D. D. Price. A physiological and psychological analysis of pain: A potential model of motivation. In Pfaff, D., Physiological Mechanisms of Motivation. New York: Springer-Verlag, 1982, 433–471.

Mecuson, R., and P. Lievens. The use of cryotherapy in sport injuries. Sports Med. 3, 398–414 (1986).

Mense, S., and R. F. Schmidt. Muscle pain: Which receptors are responsible for the transmission of noxious stimuli? In Rose, F. C. (ed), Psychological Aspects of Clinical Neurology. Oxford: Blackwell Scientific Publications, 1977, 265–278.

Pappenheimer, J. R., S. L. Eversole, and A. Soto-Rivera. Vascular response to temperature in the isolated perfused hindlimb of the cat. Am. J. Physiol. 155, 458 (1958).

Procacci, P., and M. Zoppi (eds). Pathophysiology and clinical aspects of visceral and referred pain. In Bonica, J. J., et al. (eds.), Advances in Pain Research and Therapy, vol 5. New York: Raven Press, 1979, 643–658.

Reenie, C. A., and S. D. Michlovitz. Biophysical principles of heating and superficial heating agents. In Michlovitz, S. L., Thermal Agents of Rehabilitation. Philadelphia: Davis, 1996.

Roddie, I. C., and J. T. Shepherd. The contribution of constrictor and dilatator nerves to the skin vasodilatation during body heating. J. Physiol. (Lond.) 136, 489–497 (1957).

Rubin, D. Myofascial trigger point syndromes. An approach to management. Arch. Phys. Med. Rehabil. 62, 107–110 (1981).

Scholander, P. F., H. T. Hammel, K. Lange-Andersen, and Y. Loving. Metabolic acclimatization to cold in man. J. Appl. Physiol. 12, 1–8 (1958).

Scholander, P. F., J. S. Hart, D. H. Le Messurier, and J. Stein. Cold adaptation in Australian aborigines. J. Appl. Physiol. 13, 211–218 (1958).

Selkins, K. M., and A. P. Emery. Thermal science for physical medicine. In Lehmann, J. F. (ed); Therapeutic Heat and Cold, third ed. Baltimore: Williams & Wilkins, 1982.

Selye, H. The general adaptation syndrome and the diseases of adaptation. J. Clin. Endorinol. Metab. 6, 117 (1946).

Simons, D. G., and J. G. Travell. Myofascial origins of low back pain. Postgrad Med. 73, 66 (1983).

Smith, J. D. Constriction of isolated arteries and their vasavasorum produced by low temperature. Am. J. Physiol. 171, 537–538 (1952).

Steilan, J., and B. Habot. Improvement of pain and disability in elderly patients with degenerative osteoarthritis of the knee treated with narrow band light therapy. J. Am. Geriatr. Soc. 40(1), 23–26 (1992).

Taber, C., K. Countryman, J. Fahrenbruch, et al. Measurement of reactive vasodilatation during cold gel pack application to non-traumatized ankles. Phys. Ther. 72(4), 294–299 (1992).

Travell, J. G., and D. G. Simons. Myofascial Trigger Point Manual. Baltimore: Williams & Wilkins, 1982.

U.S. Department of Health and Human Services. Treatment of Pressure Ulcers: Clinical Practice Guidelines. Rockville, MD: U.S. Department of Health and Human Services, 1994.

Wahlund, W. Determination of the physical working capacity. Acta Med. Scan. 132 (Suppl.), 215 (1948).

Walsh, M. T. Hydrotherapy: The use of water as a therapeutic agent. In Michlovitz, S. L. (ed.), Thermal Agents in Rehabilitation, third ed. Philadelphia: Davis, 1996.

Warren, C., J. Lehmann, and J. Koblanski. Heat and stretch procedures. An evaluation using rat tail tension. Arch. Phys. Med. Rehabil. 57, 122–126 (1976).

Wessman, M. S., and F. J. Kotrke. The effect of indirect heating on peripheral blood flow, pulse rate, blood pressure and temperature. Arch. Phys. Med. Rehabil. 48, 567–576 (1967).

Weston, M., C. Taber, L. Casagranda, et al. Changes in local blood volume during cold gel pack application to non-traumatized ankles. J. Orthop. Sport Phys. Ther. 19(4), 197–199 (1994).

Wolf, S. L. Contra lateral upper extremity cooling from a specific cold stimulus. Phys. Ther. 51, 158–165 (1971).

Zankel, H. T. Effect of physical agents on motor conduction velocity of the ulnar nerve. Arch. Phys. Med. Rehabil. 45, 787–792 (1966).

Zimmermann, M. Peripheral and central nervous mechanisms of nociception, pain and pain therapy: Facts and hypotheses. In Bonica, J. J., et al. (eds.), Advances in Pain Research and Therapy, vol. 3. New York: Raven Press, 1979, 3–32.

NOTES

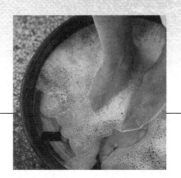